Calorie Engineering

by William Young

Dedication

For my wife Gina
and my children William, Carson, and Lucy
and my pets Marmaduke, Pebbles, Depy, and Zoe
who gave me a reason to stick around longer

For those who laughed at me when I was fat
nana nana, I am skinnier than you now

For our modern way of eating
without which this book would not be needed

Contents

Acknowledgments

Thanks to my wife, Gina, for support and helping edit. Who knew there were so many ways to misuse words?

Chapter 1: Why

"I bargained with Life for a penny, and Life would pay no more" - Jessie B. Rittenhouse

1.1. My Story

I weighed 344 pounds the day I started. Some days less; some days more. I pictured myself as overweight, but my doctor could not describe my weight with one word. It required three - very severely obese. I was in my mid-thirties, but I felt double that age in health. I hid from the future my weight was leading to. The lid blew off the hole I had hiding in after my wife and I had our first child. Would I be there with my wife, children, and dare say grandchildren one day in the future? I needed to get my weight down to one word, healthy, and I put everything I knew into it.

I was not the most athletic. Even at bowling, I came in last. I was not the smartest. Many others had higher SAT scores than me. But, I had a skill. In every facet of my life, I solved problems and accomplished whatever I focused upon. The question at work was "Which computer technology will grow sales revenue in the next five years?" In my garden, "How do I grow the world's hottest pepper?" In my garage, "How do I install a garage door opener?" Each was a delicious challenge begging for a solution, and I solved each one in turn. Yet, I never brought what I can do to bear on my weight.

Weight loss has one axiom. The calories you eat in a day decide your weight. You can get more by exercising, but calories in minus calories out mandates your weight. I ate based on the way food looked, tasted, my emotional reaction, but never calories. Salad and pizza are a world apart in calories, but I had no clue of the degree. Calories are the currency of the weight realm. Success means understanding them.

When you mention calories, people picture a life of denial. I asked, "How do I eat what I like and change the calories to fit?" Within three months, I lost over twenty pounds and no longer needed to take aspirin every day. In eighteen months, I came to the top end of healthy weight range. Another six months after that, I landed at 177 pounds, half of where I started. When I was fat, I dreamed of waking up skinny overnight. But looking back, I am glad I did not. The time I spent in getting to my current weight was an investment in being a calorie engineer. The journey was more important than my final weight. I set off to engineer the calories, which I did, but I discovered a better lifestyle.

The first day I woke up to a new lifestyle. The second day it was not as new. By the ninetieth day, the new lifestyle was mine with the old one a distant memory. I no longer understand my old self. At present, the changes are habit and I am on auto-pilot. I pay attention to calories, adjust them to my needs, and make good choices. I may still have deep-dish pizza or a large Thanksgiving dinner. But, even then I am like an experienced tightrope walker. The real win is that every day my lifestyle is one better than I could have imagined.

I have put forth what I have learned in solving my weight loss problem. It does not require an engineer's degree. Not even much math is required. If you can use a calculator, you are qualified. It requires openness to a new lifestyle. I invite you to try this program. This book was for me to look back on my journey, but now it is for you a journey I offer. The scale will not go drop twenty pounds a week after starting. Make a three month commitment and then check the scale.

I hate to admit it, but I was happy with my old lifestyle before I began. Thus, the first question to ask yourself is why do you want to change your lifestyle to lose weight? Having an answer to the why question is more important than any number on a scale.

1.2. Baking Time

When I slept, I snored like a noisy mixer. My wife told me I sat up in my sleep because I did not breathe well. After nine hours sleep, I staggered out of bed and hit the snooze button a few times. It took ten minutes to find the pet dishes, open the food cans, and feed the pets. The whole time I questioned "Why do not I feed the pets at night instead?" After that, food stayed last on my mind. It was the one time of day I could pass by leftover cake. I added one or two items or plates to lunch of dinner to make up for the missed meal.

As I lost weight, I quit snoring. My wife complained that she was not sure if I was awake or had left the room. Today I slept for seven and half hours and woke up rested. I forgot how the snooze button works and moved the alarm clock to the other side of the bedroom. When I stay up late watching the Walking Dead on Sunday night, I do not hit the snooze button the next morning. I spend the same amount of time getting ready in the morning. But I eat breakfast, feed the pets, read a few magazine articles, and start in on a work project before leaving the house.

Pizza was a food I could not live without, and none beat my homemade pizza. Yet, making a homemade pizza involved making the crust, shaping it out, baking it, cooking the sausage, putting the toppings on, and so on. Even the assembly of cooked ingredients was a major task. I only did it on the weekend. Today, pizza assembly is a weekday dinner, and I have time left over to relax from the workday.

Every spring I hauled, dumped, and arranged a pickup truck worth of mulch. I started in the morning and tried to finish by late afternoon. Last spring, I spent longer driving to pick it up and back then I did to unload it. I went back and bought a few more loads. Plus, my dogs got added exercise when they went to play in the extra mulch.

Nothing is guaranteed except chocolate in a chocolate cake. I never considered how long I would live. Death seemed far away. Whenever I wondered if being in shape would help me, I told myself I could be in great shape and get hit by a truck. That way of thinking helped me get through entire chocolate cakes. Then the plates of chocolate cake passed by and I did not feel as young.

All things being equal, I would prefer to live forever. I never want my wife and I to say goodbye to each other. But, how close I would get to forever never felt like it was in my control. It was a far out date. Far enough away not to be forced to consider it. My wife is as far away from retirement and old age as I am. To think about either of us not being there seemed too distant to worry about. It was too close to facing my mortality and I could not do that.

Then we had our first child. When he graduates high school, I will be in my fifties. I will retire from a lifelong career when he is discovering what it means to start a career. Who knows how old I will be when he has children of his own? The future spelled its way out. With decades before me, I needed to stick around for at least two more generations. I was determined to do everything for my part to ensure my time with my wife and children was as long as possible.

Each hour in a day is precious. Despite modern technology, they have not added another hour into the day. Moreover, days on this earth are limited. Time is a small serving of a chocolate cake. You always want more. Yet, I have baked the unexpected. I have gained more time. From sleeping less to being quicker, I have more hours in a day to do things. And I have done my part to improve my health, increasing my days. My slices of food may be smaller in calories, but I gained a bigger slice of time. A billionaire would mortgage away everything for more time, yet it cannot be bought. I knew time was a limited resource but did not realize I could create more. If I was talking to my old self, I would say "Sounds nice, but tell me about the food." However, the current me would pick more time over any slice of chocolate cake.

1.3. Vibrant Vitality

Whenever I came down with the flu, I fought my best to keep working through it. As long as I could still work and get things done, I did not feel that bothered by it. What frustrated me is that when I got sick, I felt like overcooked stale bread. Yet once I recovered, I felt normal, not great, and not even good. Eating became a flu. Not eating left me feeling like I had the flu. No matter how much ice cream and pizza I ate, I felt normal afterward, not great. It was like I had a perpetual flu chasing me. But, I could still carry on my life, so it did not make me take notice.

Then one day the flu feeling stayed with me. I felt bad, no matter how much I ate. I thought I was getting old. I started taking vitamins and aspirin to see if that would help. Maybe it happened one day overnight, or maybe it was gradual day by day. Either way, it came to a tipping point that I had to deal with.

Today, I can close my eyes, take a deep breath, and feel marvelous. When I get the flu, getting back that feeling is what I most look forward too. When the kids are discovering new ways to destroy the house, I understand why our ancestors lived in rock caves. At times like that, I close my eyes and take a deep breath and feel the good feeling inside.

When I was fat, I did more physical outdoor activities than most skinny people I knew through my gardening hobbies. Somebody told me I was lying to myself in saying that. I wondered if there was any truth to that. Now I am a healthy weight and I know I was not lying. I could weed a large field, arrange mulch, or anything else I wanted to do outside. My garden had more square footage than most houses. I had a tiller and ten different gardening hoes, each one for a specific situation. My tools should have allowed me to maintain a garden ten times bigger. But I started questioning if the garden was worth it or if I should reduce the size.

Every week I walked through the entire local zoo. Then one day I walked through half of it instead. Then many months later, I walked through the entire zoo again. It was harder than I remember, but I could push myself through it. The experience left me wondering if the second half of the zoo was worth the walk.

The single activity I felt caught off from was running, but I had no desire to run a marathon. If I tried to run, then I hurt for days afterward. I viewed running as something strange invited by health nuts.

Thus, I did not see anything missing in my life nor did I see lies. I burned thousands of calories in those days, but went on reward trips to the buffet. However, I understand something deeper now.

In my garden this spring, I cleared a few beds hoeing instead of a tiller to compare speed and effectiveness between the two methods. I judged which one was better. It went so fast I got carried away and ended up extending the garden even more. I now have more space to plant than plants I want to grow. This is for the best as I have children that I need to draft into helping, so I need more chores for them when they get older.

Going through the entire zoo is now a question of if the kids are ready for their nap. I would like to go through the whole zoo multiple times over, but the kids start to get cranky about halfway through. I once heard a child asking his dad to go see everything and his dad said "Do not worry. I want to go through the whole zoo and see it everything." I thought I cannot wait till my kids are older.

Now I run in the yard for the fun of it. I take off with my legs and body moving faster than ever before and feel like part of the wind. My dog runs with me. Afterward, he is panting and lays down, tired. I tell him, "I used to be like you". I may build up my stamina and enter a marathon next year.

The fat slowed me down on things, but it never stopped me from doing anything I wanted to do. Instead, it removed my desire to go through the whole zoo or keep a large garden. It did so one pound at a time without me realizing it. It is not about being able to do physical activities. Instead it was about a fog of fat clouding my mind removing any desire to do physical activities.

One of the things that scared me when my first child was born was the thought of not being able to be there for him. Kids are filled with a Peter Pan level of energy. How would I keep up with one? But now I have enough energy to not only keep up with my toddler, but to out run him and tire him out. Once we are both older, he will be able to out run me. But that is a long way off, and he is going to have to work if he wants to be able to do that. I am happy too that he will not grow up with food like I did.

Back when I felt bad, I went to see a doctor. He sent me for a well being test. I had high blood pressure, high bad cholesterol, and the results were a page of red. The test was pointless because it reflected how I knew I felt on the inside. If it had all came back as good numbers, then I would have been in trouble. This year, I retook the same tests. From blood pressure through triglycerides, I am in solid green. I did not feel like I needed that test either because I feel good.

1.4. Food Fears

Where the food would lead concerned me, frightened me, and left me reluctant to change things in the past. Yet, food does not have the grasp on me it used to, and I eat better than before. This morning I had a rainbow of flavors for breakfast. I had Greek yogurt with frozen strawberries, blackberries, and special dark cocoa. The blackberries left in the freezer are from the end of the season. That crop had a harder taste than the main middle crop. Dark chocolate cocoa brings a chocolate flavor I do not confuse with sugar. For my second course, I had two eggs fried in half a tablespoon of cream butter. These went on two slices of toasted sourdough bread made with whole wheat. As the last touch, I put two pork sausage patties on top. My whole breakfast came in at five hundred sixty calories. I did not crave to eat again until hours later at my normal lunch time.

Back when I was fat, a morning compromised four eggs, maybe five. I did not hit six eggs, or at least I think I did not. The eggs were fried in amounts of butter best described as gobs. I used at least one and often three pieces of toast and sausage patty for each egg. The bread was a store bought ancient grain of inner peace variety. It was triple the calories of normal bread, but the label said it was healthy. I drank orange juice with the meal because it was my picture of a healthy breakfast drink. A candy chaser followed the meal. I preferred milk chocolate because it has more sugar than chocolate. After that feast, I was ready to eat by the time I got to the couch.

Halloween brings back memories of getting candy from houses and learning to avoid the houses that did not give out candy. There were a few prized houses that passed out whole candy bars. I ate my booty within a few days if not within one. When Halloween rolls back around and candy is everywhere, those memories come back. A piece of candy brings back my memory of the childhood joy it used to bring. But, when I try a piece, it tastes like dirt that has been in the oven too long. I spit it out. My wife laughs at me. The next piece tastes the same way, and the one after that. I cannot believe the candy I used to enjoy tastes so bad. After two more pieces, I give up and conclude that it tastes that way now. I then need to eat something good to get rid of the bad taste, like apple crisp, which has a nice crunchy topping over sweet apples. As I eat it, I realize I never knew what was good.

In the old days, I looked for ways to layer in sugar. I made brownies with milk chocolate chips added and chocolate icing on top. Caramel fudge drop ice cream married my brownie in the bowl. Today, when I review a recipe, I ask "How can I get the calories down and have it taste good?" For instance, I make apple crisp with sweet apples, which do not need sugar added to them. Then use molasses and sucralose in the topping instead of brown sugar. And I discovered I only needed half the butter called for in the topping. I bake it in ramekins so that the serving size is defined. Apple crisp becomes calorie friendly without sacrificing flavor. When apples come in season, I buy extra and make apple crisp every other day. Through the journey, discovering new ways to optimize calories brought as much enjoyment as when I used to discover a forgotten bag of candy.

Somewhere in the pounds, my tastes changed. I do not think about ice cream with caramel fudge drops. I might sit and think apple or apple crisp. But it has been a long time since I have desired ice cream with caramel fudge drops. Most of the old desserts are like an old friend who I have lost touch with and do not seem to have anything in common. Before I could taste the level of sugar added to fruit in a dessert. Now, I can taste the different type of berries and when in the season they were harvested. I enjoy what I eat. I used to explore sugar, but now I explore food with flavor.

1.5. Not Expensive

The grocery store could afford to hire an extra person with what I spent for foods with labels proclaiming healthy. In the cereal aisle every box had a healthy check box and a prize inside. But the boxes that had real food in them were over double the ones with the plastic prize. As another example, I went through a phase of trying to eat vegetarian once a week for dinner. The processed frozen vegetarian section was the first place I turned. The food may have been vegetarian, but it was priced like steak. Even turning to lean beef was difficult. In the butcher section, the lean cuts of ground beef approached and passed the price of steak. If cereal, vegetarian, and ground beef are expensive, where did that leave healthy eating?

The produce section did not have the health labels the rest of the store offered. But, the fruits and vegetables were as cheap as the dirt they grew in. Every weekend, I purchased ten pounds of bananas. For five dollars I get enough bananas to last my family a week. It got expensive if I bought off season fruits, like fresh strawberries in winter, but that was when I turned to the frozen section. Elsewhere in the store, a pound of brown rice or dried beans were less than two dollars. Even a decent sized box of parboiled brown rice was under three dollars. In the refrigerator section, a whole chicken sells for a dollar per pound, and chicken breast for two dollars per pound. Minimally processed foods are minimally priced. Those were the foods I have built my new eating habits around. The grocery store may have had to let go of that extra person I was subsidizing, but my wallet and health are better for it.

Then there was dining out. I knew someone who said he saved up all month for an expensive dinner out with his wife. He told me about the price of the steak and wine. There was a five minute overview of how tips worked when his father-in-law was with him. During the whole time, I heard no mention of how satisfying the food was, not even a generic fresh comment. It was about the pleasure of wasting money. At those rates, it does not take long, until you cannot only afford healthy food, you can remodel the kitchen.

Meanwhile, my dragon was the drive-thru. Nothing brought home inflation more than seeing the dollar menu re-branded to the value menu. I started with a cheeseburger for a dollar. Then debate if I should add bacon for a dollar more. For a few more, I could super size the fries. The apple pie was two for a dollar. Did not I deserve an apple pie to go with it? The value menu is the gateway drug to spending on fast food. Moreover, the values are good for a single meal for a single person. Once I purchase a few value hamburgers, I have spent enough to buy the ingredients to make multiple hamburgers at home.

A decade ago, I bought a computer printer based on the best price for a good brand and features. The printer lasted a decade. In that time, I paid the price of at least two computers in buying ink. When the last fifty dollar cartridge of ink ran out, I threw out the printer. This time I asked what models had the cheapest ink? Computer printers are the poster child of why you should look at the total cost of ownership. I view food in the same way, except the ink bill does not come due as soon. When I was younger, I had no appreciation for health care costs. Today, instead of saving for retirement, I am saving for health care. One hospital visit wipes out any alleged savings from a year of the value menu.

However, better food is not worth any price. I continue to be thrifty. I use that way of thinking to make sure I am not taking false short cuts in savings. This comes in with heavily processed foods that may appear cheap.

1.6. Willpower

I tried other weight loss approaches. I was prepared to do anything except change my lifestyle. Eat all you want, but eat vegetarian. For half a year, I tried being vegetarian at least half the day. It is amazing how many good tasting vegetarian options there are from bread, olive oil, and juice. It was not that hard of a change. Despite my serious efforts, I did not lose any weight. Eat all you want, but work out. One New Year I purchased a recumbent exercise bike. I started off focused. I would look up silly questions online. Does it matter if I eat a big meal before or after I use the exercise bike? I went with after as a reward. I did not lose any weight. Next, temporarily do major cut backs on eating and lose weight. Then go back eating all you want and gain more weight back. None of these gimmicks worked for me. None asked me to make any permanent lifestyle changes. Avoiding one food and overeating everything else is not a lifestyle change. It is a different song on the radio rather than a different station. Worse, all the approaches made it seem as if you focus willpower on changing one thing.

Before I started this program, I liked my lifestyle and feared changing it. I thought it would be hard to engineer calories. I did not know what I was getting myself in for at the start. The thought of looking at the calories in the food for the rest of my life left me wondering how much of a struggle the rest of my life would be. I pictured a cage match of the donut versus me, and I knew how that had gone in the past.

The willpower ended up being the commitment to start, and that was more determination than willpower. The first month was a shift in my approach to food. I questioned if a food was worth its calories or if a recipe could be cut down in calories. In short, I began to think analytically about calories. Week over week, my lifestyle began to change a pound at a time. After a few months, thinking about calories became a regular habit, like brushing my teeth. I do not have any more willpower than when I started. If I worked in a donut factory, then that would be the end of me. However, I have better habits now. Even when I eat a donut, I eat one donut, but I used to eat half a dozen on my own. Moreover, I pick other foods over donuts.

I thought it would be willpower to create a calorie deficit. I pictured raw sea weed served on a small plate. Then I could feel myself hating every bite and forcing myself to eat it. It ended up being far from the truth. Besides better habits, I gained knowledge. I learned how to right size the calories in the foods I liked to eat. I have felt like my whole life has been about knowledge, figuring out things. It was fitting that food was the same way.

I used to look at a bowl of ice cream and think I cannot wait to eat it. Now the calories come to mind before the first bite. Moreover, I learned the different ways to slice the calories down. Drop the nuts from the ice cream and save a hundred calories. Eat a frozen banana that has been run through the food processor instead of eating ice cream and save hundreds. The calories dropped themselves once I engineered them. The journey was never about will power for me, but rather learning a new approach to food and then to my life.

1.7. Strong Reasons

Among the seven billion people on the planet, one guy holds the title of fattest person alive. I bet he thinks the second fattest guy is fatter than him. They are different heights. How do you compare? Beyond those two, fat is the growing majority in America. I can find someone fatter than me as quick as finding another fast food restaurant. Comparing myself to others is not any motivator. I was big when I started, but I am sure the laggards would have caught up in time.

A few months back I met up with old high school acquaintances I had not seen in years. It brought back memories to see them again. Some good. Some bad. But, I was delighted that even the high school hot shots grew fatter. I was the skinniest person in the group. Do they like me any better because I weigh less? Do I care? I did not impress people back in high school. I am sure not out to impress them or anyone else. This journey was for myself.

When I was younger, I had a hard time finding 2XT shirts. Today, I could go to my local clothing store and pick up a 4XT off the rack. I wondered if I would have trouble finding shirts if I grew anymore. Then I discovered online clothing stores catering to extraordinary customers such as myself. They went up several more notches. I had buffer to grow. The fashion industry is out to make money. They will keep expanding sizes with the population.

Many years back I wore an ocean blue shirt with 79 written on it with the American flag as the number background. I wore it at least once a week. When it squeezed too tight, I saved it, with other clothes, hoping one day I would fit into it again. When I started to lose weight, wearing my old clothes meant as much as any number on the scale. Once I got below three hundred, I kept asking my wife "Does this fit?" Then one day the answer was yes. It had a few holes in it and was more of a rustic blue color. Then one day it was too big and I had to quit wearing it because I will never fit into it again. The shirt had a few holes and been more bluish than blue. But, when I put it on, I felt as young as I was when it was new. Wearing those old clothes again was not enough to make me want to change my lifestyle. As much as I loved my old blue flag t-shirt, I loved a bowl of ice cream more. Still, it was a nice encouragement along the way.

Part of my obesity problem was not having a working method to lose weight. But, much of the problem is having a reason. Peter Pan could fly if he had a happy thought. I needed to find my happy thought to get me through the program. The reasons I embarked on this journey are my personal ones. To tailor for your own needs, you have to look inside and ask questions. What matters most to you? What are you afraid of losing out on? Why is the world any worse off if you are not in it tomorrow? These are tough questions, like turning down a donut tough. I said it was not a test of willpower, but maybe I am wrong.

Maybe it is the willpower to face yourself and find motivation that matters to yourself.

1.8. What Is Food?

Food was a friend to have a good time with. The kind I had wild parties with when I was younger. As a friend, it was there for me when the world shined the brightest and when I needed someone. I was not thinking food was a friend, but I acted that way. Recognizing that all food was not my friend was my first paradigm shift in thinking of food. And finding someway to think of food in the right way was the second.

I would take a vacation to Hawaii every week if it cost twenty dollars each trip. It is closer to thousands, and many people go once every few years. But what if it was the price of a house and required a thirty year mortgage? How often would you go then? Where is your cut off spending for a good time of enjoyment? When do you say I will go to the local beach instead?

Meanwhile, the turtle milkshake from the drive-thru provides two minutes of enjoyment that do not require going through airport security. But what is the calorie cost of that shake? Is it worth the calories in a three course meal? Or the calories in an entire day? Where is that calorie cut-off point? And when do you say I will substitute with a lower calorie treat? For instance, I can make a homemade shake for less than half a meals worth of calories.

In my mind, the Hawaii trip and turtle milkshake are the same question. I think in terms of spending calories. Is it worth it? What are my other options? It does not mean you never have it. As people save for the Hawaiian trip, you can plan for the turtle milkshake, if that is what you want. As for me, I will not get suckered in on a freak Hawaiian vacation at the drive-thru.

When I over ate and borrowed calories, I accumulated debt as extra weight. The interest on that extra weight translated into lower vitality. It went right back to dollars as extra costs on health care. Not an even deal for the fleeting enjoyment I had experienced. But, I did not think I had a choice. It was eat food or starve - yes or no to the turtle milkshake. A third alternative never occurred to me.

I earned every dollar I made. To get more calories means having a healthier body. You can do more exercises to build up your muscles, so that your body burns more calories every day.

Even the irony of the rich get richer and the poor get poorer holds. The more knowledge I gained and the better habits I developed, the easier the weight loss program became. Before that, I was trending to higher numbers on the scale.

When I was growing up, my uncle Bob tried to encourage me to learn about things. He said if you do not understand something someone will take advantage of you. I thought he meant in terms of fixing a car or household repair. But, that comment speaks to my whole life with food. I did not understand food and had the pounds to prove it.

People told me no one forced me to eat those cheeseburgers. The food industry did not force me, but they did their best to tempt me. Moreover, no one forced the food industry to sell processed food loaded with calories. The food industry is there for profits. They will sell whatever people will buy. Nothing more than greed. I suppose my overeating was being too greedy with food in a way. The food industry and me, two adversaries, locked in a game, both motivated by greed.

The big advantage in the game I have is the other side must disclose the calories. They will take a shake and put a Hawaiian beach label on it. Everything they can do to get you to ignore the calories. Yet, food is labeled with the calories or can be looked up online.

The food industry will appeal to anything that helps you feel better about their food. Concerned on carbs? No problem, we have tons of high calorie foods that are carb free. Concerned on fat? More good news. All products derived from pure sugar are fat free. Enjoy. Vegetarian, GMO free, the Easter bunny, and everything else is used as a marketing gimmick. They even try to deceive the amount of sugar added by adding different forms of sugar, so that sugar will not be the first ingredient in the list. The pursuit of money has evolved the food industry into efficient super-marketers. They know our weaknesses and will do their best to exploit them. Until you gain the knowledge that my uncle Bob talked about, you cannot win against them.

It stings like a bee to compare overeating to an addiction like smoking. There is a clear outcome to a smoking habit. Quit smoking.

Never have another cigarette. I do not smoke, but I understand the desired outcome. Take overeating, which I did, what is the desired outcome? It is not to quit eating, not even to quit particular groups of foods. The desired outcome is to eat the right amount, no more, no less. Could you picture telling a smoker he has to find the right amount of cigarettes to smoke in a day? And that the right number was specific to him?

Despite the end goal difference, there are similarities. Smoking has control over the people who do it. It is not a habit easily kicked. Food had control over me, and my eating habits were not changed easily. There are many ad campaigns against second hand smoke. But, there is a form of second hand overeating. I feel better over indulging on food when I do with someone else. Then I think about role models for my kids. I would not want them seeing me as a role model smoking or overeating.

The anti-obesity ad campaign is as useful as replacing anti-smoking with anti-lung cancer. It does not speak to the cause. A restaurant can market a milkshake that has a day's worth of calories. The majority of people derail others for pointing that out. I used to be one of them doing the derailing. Yet, cigarettes have poison labels on them. If you smoke, you accept it is bad for you because there is no avoiding the ad campaigns. Yet when I overeat, I can lie to myself because there is no equivalent ad campaign. I have never seen a poison label on any food in the grocery store, even though many deserve the label. The obesity campaign focuses on the after fact and not the food at cause. The key in the smoking comparison was for me to gain control over myself as anyone else with an addiction must do.

Chapter 2: Food Journal

"Annual income twenty pounds, annual expenditure nineteen six, result happiness. Annual income twenty pounds, annual expenditure twenty pound ought and six, result misery." - Charles Dickens, David Copperfield

2.1. Why Journal

Years back, I heard pop was bad for my weight, so I switched to juice. It seemed healthier. But juice can have as many or more calories than pop. I knew a milkshake was high in calories, but I had no relative concept of how many compared to a hamburger, a side of fries, or even a salad. Yet, I still gained every pound that made me obese. Ignorance was not bliss; it was obesity. My body was pushed too far with fat to give me signals on eating enough on my own. The one signal left was when my stomach could not hold anymore food, and even that signal I ignored. As I came down in weight, my body began to work better, but I could not trust it when I was obese.

I tracked the calories in what I ate. Learning a donut is three hundred calories was more horrific than any horror movie I have ever seen. I used to eat three or more donuts in one sitting. Also, how is it that a large meat lover's pizza can have over a full days worth of calories?

Life did not seem fair. I kept reminding myself that the point was to learn, not judge.

The act of logging food gave me clues of where I could cut calories. There were small but re-occurring ones, like the cheese on the hamburger. Then there were the heavy hitters, like the ice cream after the hamburger. And the surprises, like the mayo I mentioned. My food journal started to the provide insight into which foods to emphasize and then it provided comparisons. I learned I ate less in ice cream than donuts, so I could save calories with that alone.

At first, it was easy to judge myself by what I logged and how many calories it was. That is why people quit paying attention to calories. It is scarier than any horror movie. But I soon took a different view. All those calories meant I had lots of opportunities for wins. If I had started my food journal and saw nothing that upset me, it would have been hard to make any cuts. Looking back, if I had not been eating so many high calorie foods, this would have been much harder because I would not have been able to make cuts anywhere. But seeing the donut and ice cream calories bother me meant I had some directions of where I could recover calories. A food journal is a tool, like a calculator, not a judge.

2.2. Tracking Tools

For the first ten months, I tracked my calories with a pen and paper. I kept a table going the whole day of item, amount of calories, and running calorie total. Writing it down with a pen connected me to the calories in a way I have never felt. Typing 300 or 30 is the same effort. But, writing it down and then hand adding it comes out as a different experience. Every 300 calorie donut felt painful to write and add in. In contrast, every light turkey sandwich left with me joy when I still had calories left over.

This morning I ate the same thing for breakfast as yesterday. I used my mobile app to copy yesterday's breakfast. For lunch, I entered bread. It suggested adding turkey, mayo, and the other items I eat with bread. It was faster than I ever was with my pen and paper, and I had no math errors. But, I had to pay attention to the line item calories because the difference between it is the same effort to add an apple as a donut. I make sure to read the calories entered per item and pay attention to my running total as I go along. This is the biggest risk in the mobile app. Convenience may lure you into complacency, so be sure to pay attention.

I tried to expand my paper table to track protein and other items. The complexity grew, and I felt deterred from both the work it took to track it and having to pay attention to another number. That was dangerous. If it is hard, then I knew I would not succeed. Thus, I scaled back to focus on calories. In the start, that is the single metric. I did a few rough calculations on the other nutrients. Protein powered my meals - no worries there. For the vitamins, I took a multivitamin as an insurance against missing any of them in my pursuit of lowering calories. Other than that, I saw nothing else I needed to pay attention to. My primary goal was to master calories and lose weight.

A mobile app makes it trivial to track protein, fat, carbs, and everything else. It has nice reports about how I averaged out over the past week. Even when I used the mobile app, I ignored those reports. Once I was no longer obese, I paid attention to the vitamins and other nutrients. I had many months in by that point, so I felt comfortable with the calories. Since I pursued less processed lower calorie foods, I was doing well. I quit taking the multivitamin. I swam in vitamin C but not as much vitamin A. Foods like carrots and plantains are higher in vitamin A. I made efforts to add them into my eating. Once you master the calories, you can go on to other metrics to the degree you desire.

I often did not have my paper log with me when I was out of the house or traveling. I had to make a note and remember to log when I got back home. My normal weekday was to eat breakfast before leaving, eat lunch at work, and then eat dinner at home. Thus, I only had to remember lunch. I tended not to snack in the day at work. It was more of a minor pain than a major failing. The big risk is forgetting to add something.

I do not have even that minor pain with my cell phone. I carry around my smart phone like it is attached to me. When I eat something, I can add it into my cell phone. That is the most ideal time. I was good at keeping my paper journal up to date, but removing the risk with my cell phone helped tilt me to using it instead.

Then there are other features that my paper journal cannot match. When I pick up a container of mayo, I can scan the bar code into my food journal. I do not even have to type to add what I am eating. Plus, the mobile app has a large database of food information. Rather than search the web, I can search in the app and find what I am looking for. And mine is hooked into tracking the steps I walk with my phone and adds back in the calories. That feature made me put down my pen in favor of a mobile app.

A mobile app helps with goal setting. I entered my height, weight, and how much I wanted to lose per week. Then it calculated how many calories I should eat each day. As the day progresses, it tells me how many calories I have left. I enjoy this feature, but I will mention two caveats. First, like the calorie entry, the difference between two pounds per week and a half pound per week is a click away. Be careful on setting unrealistic goals. They will derail you. I discuss this later in the book. Second, the particular app I use re-adjusts my daily calories every time I update my weight. I do not want my calories adjusted every time the scale moves. There is not any stability or getting used to a calorie level. Thus, I tended to update my weight every few weeks, even if I weighed myself more often. Side benefit, the weight loss graph looks like a smooth road instead of the jagged mountain path it was. I figured out how to override it and set an explicit number of calories. I recommend doing the same.

There is another journal method I tried but do not recommend. I am a long-term computer nerd. My first attempt was a custom spreadsheet on the computer instead of paper. I customized it with all the food metrics. I pulled in advanced spreadsheet functions, like pivot tables and VLOOKUP function. I got as much enjoyment out of playing with the spreadsheet as eating. But, it was not useful in practice. There were only so many things you can do with a graph of vitamin C consumed per hour. Plus, going to the computer to update my food journal every time I ate was a chore like washing the dishes after eating. By contrast, my paper and phone were right on the kitchen table. There is still fun I have with a spreadsheet of my food journal, but it is not my record.

Overall, I recommend finding a good mobile app and using that. You might need to try multiple ones to compare to find one you like.

Simplicity is the most important factor. The various features are nice, but remember to emphasis calorie tracking. As with me, you may find your method or app changes as you progress in the journey. If keeping track of calories is a chore, try a new app. I went through several mobile apps for calorie tracking. A bad one will work against you. Do not be afraid to break up with it and try a new one.

2.3. Journal Mechanics

When I ate my first hamburger under this program, I looked up the calories for everything in it. Lettuce had fifteen calories per five cups, so I figured I was using less than a calorie. I used five calories worth of onion. Neither felt important to log. If I run over my calorie goal by six calories, then that is still a success. When I use a whole tomato, it costs twenty calories, so I add it. Whenever I was in doubt, I added the food. Lettuce, onions, and other five calorie items I did not bother entering. Five is the threshold for calorie free labels. Anything less than five calories can legally be labeled as zero calories. Thus, that threshold seemed good for me.

Once I was out of the obese range, I recorded the onions and peppers. But, not for calories because by that point I looked at my overall nutrients. A pepper is loaded with vitamin C. Doing so helped me learn the other nutrients in the vegetables I eat and how I was doing on them.

What is more important is to look up and know what is important. I expected lettuce to be low, but it surprised me by how low it was. I thought the mayo would be low too. It turned out I would need a five gallon bucket of lettuce and onions to begin to equal the calories in mayo. The majority of calories in my hamburger were from the bun, the mayo, and the meat - in that order. Likewise, I discovered the calories in my side salad were coming from the salad dressing, not the salad.

Drinks are easy to forget to log. One of my first changes in eating was to switch to zero calorie drinks with my meals, like diet pop, water, and tea. Thus, I did not need to worry about logging calories from drinks. However, if I was still drinking full calorie beverages, like pop or juice, then I would have been logging those too.

I update my food journal as I eat. If I wait until the end of the day, then I forget. It can be manageable when I am away at work for the day and if no one brought in treats. Long term, it becomes tougher, as food is everywhere. Even at work, people bring in donuts, bagels, and other food. But my mobile app is with me everywhere.

There are days when my cell phone battery dies or I forget it. One those days, when I am trying to recall the whole day of eating, I go through a list of questions. What main meals did I have? The more scheduled my eating habits became the easier that was. Were there snacks between the meals? Did I spend a few coins at the vendor machine? Anyone bring in treats? Does my emergency candy bar stash need a refill? Also, if you find this becomes a trend of having to enter everything at the end of the day, then you need to find a simpler food journal method. One that encourages you to update as you eat.

Most days, I enter the food as I go through the day. I keep a rough calories per meal goal in my head, but otherwise do not calculate the entire day in advance. However, on those days where I am planning a large item later in the day, like cake or deep dish pizza, then I take a different tack. I use my food journal as a what if calculator. I enter a day in advance. What if I use less peanut butter in my sandwich for lunch, how many slices of pizza can I have? This is helpful planning for large meals later in the day. The single caution is not to be carried away with it. It is too far to be running what if scenarios about a chicken sandwich.

The food journal is the record of what I eat, so I do not have another record to audit it. However, I found a few ways to cross check to make sure it is in the right ballpark. First, I check my grocery receipt each week. If I see cookies and ice cream on the receipt, but none in my food journal, then I know there is a gap. Moreover, I ask if the receipt list is the kind of food I want to eat. It is hard to eat right if you are buying high processed high calorie foods. Second, I check over my kitchen staples to see what I have been eating. The bag of rice getting smaller is a good sign. But if the bag of potato chips is half way gone from last week, then that is a bad sign. Third, I check over my bank register for any dining out charges. I can see how many times each month I get pizza out, and how many times I am eating at high calorie restaurants. None of these provide a perfect audit, but are good cross checks.

2.4. Calorie Sources

The calories are labeled on most food in the grocery store. In the past, the calorie info was like the ad on a web page. Something I filter out of my sight without thinking. But, the calories were easy to find, once I looked for them. Moreover, my mobile app can add the item by scanning its bar code. That leaves me with estimating the number of servings I ate.

Raw produce, like bananas, and often anything from the butcher case, like chicken breast, are not labeled with calories. The USDA nutritional database has standard entries for those foods and others. It is better than the packaged food labels. It offers multiple serving sizes, such as a small apple, large apple, cup of apples, and hundred grams of apples. Likewise, my mobile app makes quick work out of adding those. It comes up in the recent food list after typing the first few letters of the name.

Some of the meals from a box, like Mac and Cheese, come with both a what is in the box calorie and a prepared calorie count. The prepared calorie count is if you follow their directions, adding what they suggest. I may make it higher or lower. For instance, cereal boxes are laughable because the prepared count is listed with skim milk. When I ate store-bought cereal I was using whole milk or two percent milk. Now I use unsweetened almond milk. Likewise, some of the skillet meals list adding ground beef. I substitute ground turkey and save calories. When I make substitutions, I use the box calories and then adjust for how I changed it. If I go through the trouble of substituting ingredients, I want credit for the calories.

The better I became at calorie engineering, the less likely the food had a bar code to scan. Chicken breasts, potatoes, beef, and so on do not have food labels. Thus, I searched for calories in basic foods. There are many sites out there with calorie information. The mobile app I use has an encyclopedia's worth within it including the USDA nutritional database and other users. It helps me get a result. When I get multiple results, I prefer the USDA listings. They have the meats, produce, vegetables, and more. They even have entries you should never need, like fried chicken with the breading removed after frying, for the semi-calorie conscience. When there is not something in the USDA, or there are multiple USDA results, I try to take what is in the middle range. I see chicken breast listed anywhere from twenty to sixty calories per ounce. Within that range, there will be more results clustered around a common number. As I have gone along, I get a feel for relative calories. For instance, if chicken breast comes back more than beef, then I know something is wrong with the entry.

When I do not get an exact match for what I am searching, I make the best guess I can. First, I try looking for foods close to it. Some exotic form of pizza is still in the same ballpark as pizza. Second, I try to look for the main ingredients and adjust from there. I know a pizza gets most of its calories from the breading, cheese, and toppings. Third, if all else fails, log a number any number depending on your reaction. Popcorn at local movie theaters falls into this last bucket. I do not know if the size is comparable to some of the chains that have calories listings, or if they use more or less butter. I do not have popcorn at the theater that often to fret too much over it. The more I have gone along, the better I get at not having to make guesses, and making better ones when I do.

I had trouble finding good nutrition information for pulled pork after cooking. The USDA listed cooked pulled pork in BBQ sauce. But, I used a low calorie BBQ sauce and wanted calorie credit. I looked up the nutrition info for a few BBQ restaurants for straight pulled pork and used their entry.

Meat and poultry have a difference between raw calories and cooked calories. The food does not gain calories in cooking unless you add oil. Rather, cooking loses water weight, so what was four ounces cooks down to three ounces. Often raw meats are listed as calories per four ounces, and cooked meats are listed as calories per three ounces. If you are looking for something and see a large discrepancy that can be why. Be sure you are using the right one.

For homemade recipes, I add up all the ingredients and divide by the number of servings. My mobile app has a recipe feature that lets me enter the ingredients, and it does the math to calculate per serving calories. Unless I tweak the recipe, I need to enter it once.

Another option would be to find a boxed food version or restaurant version of the recipe. I do not like that one because then I get no credit for any lower calorie substitutions I do. But if you are at the start of your journey where you are more starting to track than to change things, then consider using this to start with. One other side tip, you will find many people's homemade recipes entered online too. When I searched for some of my favorite cookbook recipe, I found others had entered them. You might just try searching and seeing.

Not every meal can be home cooked. When I go out to a restaurant, I try to find a good one. A good restaurant has the calories labeled on the menu. One of my favorite Mexican restaurants labeled the calories on the menu next to the picture of the item. Even though I had eaten there countless times before, I never noticed the numbers below each picture until I paid attention to calories. The first time I dined in after starting, the menu told me the calorie difference between a burrito and enchilada. I feel at ease before ordering and after eating because I do not have to wonder how many calories I ate.

A second rate restaurant is one where the calories are posted online. I expect this from a pizza parlor since I am ordering it online. But I am disappointed at the dine-in restaurant that makes me have to go online. When I end up at one of these places, I pull up their online calorie info while ordering.

A third rate restaurant is one where there is not calorie information available online. The other two classes of restaurants get my business. I do not like feeling uncertain about what I eat. A small locally owned restaurant may have trouble in maintaining a full list. I feel uneasy in saying that. I calculate the calories in my homemade recipes and know it is not hard. But it is a slap in the face for large chain restaurants. This makes me feel like they have something to hide. Still, I try a new place or meet up with others somewhere new to me and discover there is not calorie information available. When that happens, I look up a comparable item at one of their competitors. Then I think if I had eaten there, I would not have to wonder.

Whenever I dine out, my cell phone is as important as my fork. Even if the menu is labeled with calories, I need to add together the options for the entrées and sides. When it is not listed on the menu, I have to go online and check the calories. I have checked friend's online posts at the dinner table. Calorie research is a productive use by contrast.

2.5. How to Measure

When I made my first hamburger under this program, the mayo jar said a serving was one tablespoon. I used one of my measuring tablespoons to scoop out a serving. Then I tried to put it on the bread. It was as much fun as trying to get the last drops out of a ketchup bottle. After trying to spread it out, I ended up with more of a smear where it had landed. I had to scoop out a few more tablespoons and try to guess. That left me wondering if it was practical to measure it out. The ketchup was less than twenty calories per serving, so I would not have felt bad about it. But, the mayo was seventy calories per serving. The difference of a few servings amounts to ice cream calories.

For the next hamburger, I tried a different approach. The mayo jar said fourteen grams right next to one tablespoon. I put my plate with bread on a digital kitchen scale. I used a butter knife to spread mayo across the bread adding mayo until I hit fourteen grams. Next, I hit reset on the scale and measured out the ketchup in grams. Another reset for each additional item I added. Unlike the first hamburger, it did not take longer to assemble it than to eat it. Plus, no extra dishes to wash. From then on, I used the weight measurement whenever I can. My digital kitchen scale is used more than my blender, food processor, and mixer put together.

However, I found almond milk did not say the serving size in weight. It pours out easily in a measuring cup, but I hate having to dirty another dish. I weighed it out a few times and found a cup of almond milk is about two hundred fifty grams. From then on, I placed my bowl on the scale, weighed out the granola, reset, and then poured the almond milk into the bowl until it hit the right number of grams.

I have done the same thing for sugar and other foods I eat often. I have two exceptions. First, most kitchen scales will not measure down to a teaspoon of salt. Second, if it is something I do not eat often, like pancake syrup, then I do not brother learning the weight.

If a batch of taco filling weighs one pound two and half ounces, then how do I divide that up into eight servings? I have to go get my calculator. First, I have to convert it to ounces and then divide it by number of servings. However, if the weight is five hundred twenty five grams, then there is one math problem. Moreover, I can round off the grams and divide in my head if I do not feel like reaching for the calculator. It is one step, but repeated every day. Anything that makes keeping track of food easier is worthwhile.

When I make a pizza, I spread out the sauce, toppings, and cheese. I judge by eyesight if it is distributed evenly. Then I do not weigh it by the slice. I cut it into eight slices and call it eight servings. I do the same for trays of lasagna and cupcakes. Anytime it feels like it is roughly equal per unit. But, if I have any doubts, I weigh it. For instance, my homemade buns can vary by sixty calories each one, so I weigh them. That and I like to feel the joy of getting bonus calories by removing a few crumbs.

However, how do you divide a pot of beef stew into eight servings? First, I only have to weigh a few times. If I make the recipe the same way, then it comes out about the same weight each time. Any variance is ketchup level calories. I have lost track of the last time I have weighed a batch of mashed potatoes and I make them twice or more a month. But, that only helps after you have weighed it a few times. You still have to do the initial weighing.

If the batch is small enough, then I divide it into bowls and approximate each bowl filled about the same. I like to cook in batches big enough to have leftovers for dinner the next day, so I do not use this method that often for dinner. But it works well for lunch sized servings or when I make the food in a Ramekin or muffin pan.

I weighed beef stew as I took out of the cooking pot. This means weighing what others use, like my toddler, so I can keep a running total. But you do not have to do it bowl by bowl. I weigh out a large bowl at a time and everyone can take from that. As long as I have one prior weigh-in recorded, I know the approximate calories. Thus, I can guide myself on how much to eat during the meal. Then once it gets to the end, there is less to weigh out. I did this method most of the time on this program because it was easy to start with.

Then a few months ago, my wife bought new dishes that came with serving bowls. I am glad we did not have those before because I know I would have eaten whole cartons of ice cream in them at once. My preferred method now is to put it in one large serving dish and weigh it all up front for less math and hassle during the meal. Afterward, I put the large serving bowl in the freezer for an hour or two to cool down before putting in the fridge. That was easier than in the past trying to cool down six regular sized bowls of beef stew and arrange in the fridge.

I have weighed out mayo enough times now I can approximate it. I know that one serving of mayo is a light glaze across two pieces of bread. There should not be any hills and there may be a few bare spots on the bread. The visual is perfect in my mind. I can only do this after weighing it out every day over months. However, I generally measure. I am concerned I may slip up and become more liberal on calling it a serving. I do not trust myself yet; I might one day. It is not more trouble as I am already weighing the other things I am adding to the plate.

If ice cream was 100 calories per ninety grams and I had 120 calories left, then I did the math to find out how many grams I could eat without going over. Today, I am more comfortable about ending each day over or under my calorie goal. I view my calorie goal as a range. When faced with that same dilemma today, I would either end the day under by twenty calories, or add in another half serving and be over by thirty calories. Either amount is not enough to worry about. It has been over a year since I did any per gram calculation to target an exact calorie amount.

Chapter 3: Making a Plan

"In preparing for battle I have always found that plans are useless, but planning is indispensable." - Dwight D. Eisenhower

3.1. Weight Goals

As 2014 came to a close, thoughts of hitting 199 pounds by New Years weighed on my mind. But long before then, when I started the first day, I wondered what would I have to see to know this was working? My weight fluctuated by two or more pounds from one week to the next. Thus, any small moves like going from 344 to 339 would not sell me. I thought about what would be a victory and looked down to the next weight range. I set my sights on 329. That was a weight where I could feel progress. The next question was how long to give it. At one pound per week that would be about three months. Thus, I committed to starting and seeing where I was after three months.

When I left the 330s behind, the doubts went with them. Then I became focused on 320, then 310. I aimed for multiples of five and ten as I rode the scale down. Once I made more progress, I made further goals like 290 for three months out. Each trip to the scale, I had a place I was heading in the next few weeks and the next few months.

Back at 344 it would have been a dream to wake up skinny. But I came to view that as dangerous. If I could lose it overnight, then that meant I could gain it back overnight. Taking time to hit ideal weight was insurance against reverting to obesity. The longer it took to lose it, the longer it would take to regain it. I had many pounds to go, but that meant it would take longer, not that I had to rush to lose.

As I dropped the first fifteen pounds, I realized not only did the program work, but I could ride the program down to whatever weight I desired. It might take years to get there, but it was achievable. Thus, I asked myself the question they ask you in job interviews - "Where do you see yourself in five years?" The answer was at an ideal weight, but I did not know what that number was. It was there for me, somewhere on the other side of the scale dial. I had to find it.

Body Mass Index (BMI) is measure of body fat based on weight, height, gender, and age. To calculate the number, see the appendix or my website http://WilliamRayYoung.com. The index number it provides fits into categories of how fat you are. It, like everything else in life, is an estimate. The most common objection to this scale makes me laugh. BMI does not take muscle ratio into account. Thus, a body builder shows as obese on the BMI scale. Alas, if you are reading this book, then this is not you. We are regular old fat people, and the BMI scale, while imperfect, is a useful guide to weight ranges.

A BMI score of below 25 is the top end of healthy weight. I did the math for myself, and it showed that I needed to be at 188 or less. Standing on a scale northeast of 300 and talking about weighing 188 is talk they commit you for. But I knew that was the answer to my question of where did I want to be in five years? At first, I told no one of this goal, not even my wife. Losing two pounds per week, it would take over a year. But, two pounds per week is hard to maintain for a full year. Thus, I knew the ideal weight might take every day of that five year goal, and I reminded myself of that time line whenever I wanted to go faster.

It is not like I can order clothes for a year out, and I did not think about my ideal weight each trip to the scale. My ideal weight goal was there to remind me of where my journey should take me towards. Not that I would get there on any upcoming scale visit. Each week and month, I focused on the range I was in. I never obsessed over a goal months out. Doing so would have depressed me and may have put me off the program.

For my past goals, the end date was a finish by date. If I completed it before the date, I marked it complete, forgot about it, and moved on to the next interest. I wanted this goal to be different. Thus, I set my long term goal as a future date weigh in. In November 2018, I will step on a scale and be ideal weight. Even if I hit healthy weight before then, the goal remains November 2018. When I set it up that way, it helped me think of the goal as not a due date, but a way of living. That was the motivator of ideal weight. At first I was in it to lose a few pounds, but then I wanted to make a lasting lifestyle change.

When December 2014 began, 199 by year's end did not look like it was in the scale that month. I could have achieved it if I cut my calories even further. The temptation was there, but New Years is a date. Other than that day, I was never bothered by setting specific dates. I used a rough number of weeks or months, making goals for a few weeks or a few months. I rolled into 2014 at 205, but on January 21st, I came in at 199 pounds. Looking back, I made the right choice. My life would not be different if I had hit my current weight twenty one days sooner. Focusing on the calories each day made my life different for the better.

3.2. Questions to Ask

Where does weight loss come from? The weight loss gimmicks suggest it comes from a pill, exercise, special food, or anything else that was outside of me and beyond my control. In truth, it comes from inside of me, my own body. I am not a battery like in the science fiction classic Matrix movie, but I am a calorie furnace. My body burns calories to keep the lights on. The more fat, the more calories needed. If I eat more than my body burns, then the surplus is made into more fat. If I eat less than what my body burns, then fat is burned off to cover the difference.

The essence of my weight loss approach was to eat fewer calories than my body burned doing nothing. It was a cosmic truth, like $E=MC^2$ - simple and full of power. Everything I needed to lose weight was within me and under my control. Moreover, it meant I needed to eat fewer calories, which is different than eating less food. I enjoy eating food. I do not care about eating calories. The distinction opened up techniques, and I discuss those more in the next chapter.

How many calories do I burn doing nothing? Using math similar to BMI calculations, I can estimate how many calories my body burns doing nothing each day. See the appendix or my website for the math. A good mobile app should have calorie estimation built in. To give an example, I was burning over four thousand calories each day to maintain my starting weight. Your number will be different, but will still be in thousands. The bigger the number, the more room for opportunity.

How fast can I lose weight? The better question would be how to start the weight loss journey. A half pound per week is fine to start with. But how fast was one of my burning questions at the start. The recommendation is up to one percent of your weight per week. For the fabulous fat like me, over 300 pounds, one percent per week meant three pounds per week. As I became one of the regular fat, in the 200s, this meant two pounds per week. It may not sound like much. But even one pound a year means losing fifty pounds with two weeks vacation for birthday and holidays. Many jobs do not offer that much vacation. Some weeks I wanted to lose two pounds, but only lost a pound. Some weeks the scale stayed the same; some it went up. Through it all, I kept changing my lifestyle a single day at a time.

How long will it take? The difference to the last question is important. I wanted to lose 160 pounds to get to healthy weight. That did not change how fast I could lose weight each week. I still held to the one percent of my body weight per week. Over the long term, this does mean in the one to two pounds per week range. At the start, take the weight and divide by one pound for a rough number of weeks.

How to connect weight loss goals to calorie goals? Food does not come labeled with weight loss goals. See the appendix, your mobile app, or my website http://WilliamRayYoung.com for the exact math. But as an example, if you want to lose a pound per week, then that is 3,500 fewer calories each week. That means 500 fewer calories each day. But even for the aspiring calorie engineer, we are people, not numbers. Thus, a calorie range is better than an exact number.

3.3. Daily Stop Lights

If the intersection light is green, I keep going. I stop on red. If yellow, then the decision is mine. Once I fit my calories into a stop light, they clicked in my head.

I take the calories I burn in a day doing nothing then subtract my calorie deficit. That number is my daily calorie goal. This is the green light on the stop light - my target each day. In the early days I set lots of goals, but had trouble living up to them. This is expected at first. I started with lofty weight loss goals, but had to make them into reality. It takes experience on dialing into a reasonable calorie goal. If you cannot hit the goal at least half the week, then you need to adjust and re-balance your calories across the whole week.

I thought my calorie goal was a matter of getting used to and will power. I learned it was more a matter of exploiting your engineering skills. How can I eat and be content, but with fewer calories? That is what the techniques chapters are later in this book. Your ability to do that should influence your green calorie goal.

During the week, my wife and I look forward to watching the Walking Dead on Sunday night. Then the main characters are attacked, and I am wondering how they will survive. Then the dog has to go out. The pause on the DVR comes to the rescue. There are moments in life when I need to pause what I am doing, including a calorie plan. The top limit of calories to eat in a day is the number of calories that you need to keep your current weight. Thus, no calorie deficit applied for that day. Hitting my target weight a few days later than otherwise was acceptable.

Over the years, I went from a 2x shirt to a 4x shirt. How did that happen? The truth is, I was gaining weight over the years. If I had been able to stay at 2x, then I would not have needed to lose half my body weight. The younger me did not need a weight loss program as much as a do not gain anymore weight program. The keep your current weight calories provides that victory.

I kept hitting my maintain calories in the early weeks because my original goals were too aggressive. When I over exert one day, I want to eat more the next. If I spike every few days, I smooth out the calories over every day in the week. Slow and steady wins the weight loss program. I learned through trial and error what a reasonable calorie goal was. As I pursued the calorie goal, I learned more techniques to make it possible. This let me lower overruns to two days per month, and then later onto two days per six months. It is like a TV show, a few pauses are fine, and may make the experience last longer. But a TV show filled with non-stop pauses is not enjoyable.

On the first day of a one of my college classes, the professor asked everyone what grade they wanted for the class. My reaction was that I was aiming for an A-grade, but the question was not fair. I did not know how interesting the class would be, what else would come up in my life, and how well of a teacher he was. Walking away with a B-grade was not my goal, but was something I would never give a second thought. That is like my yellow calorie goal. Somewhere between my ideal calorie deficit goal and my maintain weight calories I am fine and comfortable. If you are not sure, divide the difference between the two in half and call that your yellow calorie goal.

At a daily yellow amount I was not burning as much as I wanted. This will make things go slower. But, who cares if it takes more weeks or months? I may not have burned as much as I wanted, but I was still having a calorie deficit and still contributing to my weight loss goal. It took me a year and half to get to the top end of healthy weight. I would still have a story if it took me a full five years.

Early on I was yellow most days. I started with too aggressive of a goal, but I made progress.

When I exceed my weight calories, I feel sick and want to eat more the next day. But, I did get the enjoyment of eating. When I eat too little, I feel run down and want to eat more the next day. Yet, I get none of the enjoyment of eating. If I had to choose between being over or under by a thousand calories, then I would pick over on calories. Granted it is not a scenario I have ever faced, but it illustrates my feelings. During this program, it scared me more to go too much under calories.

As long as I am not going over calories every day, then I could still recover. My overall weight loss would take longer. Time is the one thing that is plentiful. Falling off the wagon is not a problem if you know there is a wagon that works.

The danger of going under is it takes away the wagon. This book supplies the techniques on how to create a calorie deficit. The other point of failure is this: Too aggressive of a goal makes you quit. Many years before, I dabbled with paying attention to calories for two days. I learned you cannot go from four thousand calories per day to one thousand per day.

Food is not there to keep you fat although it seems that way. Each day, your body needs vitamins, nutrients, and fresh calories. What adds further insult is that when your calories are too low, your body thinks you are out in the wild starving to death. It then kicks into calorie conservation mode, slows down your metabolism, and saves every single calorie that it can. This defeats any help from starving yourself.

The smallest recommendation is 1,200 calories per day for women and 1,500 calories per day for men. But if you are starting obese, your minimum needs to be at least double that. For me, I took it as 200 calories below my targeted calorie deficit and tried to get closer if I could.

At first, it felt like someone else controlled the stop lights. But now the stop lights are part of my thinking and are run by me. Trying to reach my calorie goal being green, with an in-between acceptable amount being yellow, and maintain current weight being red. I thought of the too little calories as driving the wrong way. In the start, you will have to adjust to realistic goals. There will be jumps. But, once you are adjusted you should hit your ideal calorie deficit most of the time.

3.4. Planning the Day

For my prior life, I ate when I walked past food, when someone offered food, when my stomach was not stuffed, when I was happy, when I was sad, and when I was indifferent. The only thing that did not drive my eating was a plan of when I wanted to eat.

Before this program, I realized how I was eating throughout the day. I reasoned if I ate fewer times in the day, I would lose weight. I avoided breakfast as it gave me more time to sleep. I skipped lunch because I thought it would let me get more done at work. Then I would have a large dinner with ice cream after. Despite sticking to that plan for months, my reasoning proved off, and I gained weight as if I had been eating more meals. When I started this program, I set out to structure my eating and looked to the classic guide of breakfast, lunch, and dinner to guide me.

I make each meal my own and turn it into a key part of my day beyond the food. On the weekdays, I leave for work before my family is up. Breakfast is my quiet time to read a magazine over a bowl of yogurt. As I eat, I pause to finish reading sections that caught my interest. The reading helps pace out the meal. On the weekends, I make bread dough or a batch of granola in the morning. I pace these out between my different breakfast items, like yogurt and then fried eggs after starting the bread dough in the mixer. For lunch, it is a few minutes break in a day of urgent items. For dinner, I make it a family dinner. My oldest may complain he is done before I start eating, but rounding up the family in the attempt of a family dinner is still my goal. My after dinner snack is after the kids go to bed and is time for my wife and I to connect. They are not meals, but rather posts of my day. Missing one of those means my routine for the day is off, which is different than saying I am not going to eat a meal because I am busy.

Breakfast and lunch were tough to squeeze in. At breakfast time, I wanted to hit the snooze button, not wake up and eat. As I lost weight and slept better, this problem went away. At first, I would suggest trying to keep a schedule as best as you can, but know once you make some progress, breakfast will be easier to fit in. Meanwhile, lunch can be challenging. The middle of the day is an opportune time for meetings. The urgent morning items have been replaced by the must finish for the day items. That challenge is why I skipped or neglected it, but now I fight to squeeze in at least five minutes. It does not have to be elaborate. And if I am in meetings in the middle of the day, I will eat during one or step out in the middle of one. Once I started trying, I can fit lunch in typically now more than a half hour from when I normally take it. On the weekends, I have found a special challenge with lunch. It takes until ten o'clock to get the family up and ready to go, which is not that far before lunch. If we are going to go somewhere, I will delay the trip or eat half a lunch before we go. I cannot say I ever had trouble fitting in dinner.

I avoid high sugar items in my meals. For breakfast, lunch, and dinner, I am looking for a meal of multiple items that is high in protein, good fat, and non-sugar carbs. Food that is high in all three is ideal. I began with store bought breakfast cereal and was ready for lunch when I got to work. That stuff is no better than eating sugar sprinkles for breakfast. Greek yogurt, fried eggs, french toast, homemade granola, and many others are my breakfast now. When I have to go work, it was hard to pull off a good lunch because it used to mean going to a drive-thru. The drive-thru tacos were high in sand, but not much else. In contrast, a peanut butter sandwich nails every macro nutrient in my list and is easy to take to work. Even for my after dinner snack, I try not to put in too much sugar, so that I do not burn out before bed. For instance, my homemade chocolate cake for four uses two tablespoons of sugar.

Each meal is the same ballpark of calories day to day. I started with dinner being the largest, breakfast being the smallest, and only an after dinner snack if I happened to have left over calories. Overtime, breakfast became my second largest meal. Dinner is still my largest, but only by about a hundred or two calories more than breakfast or lunch. And after getting into the habit of eating the same amount, I reserve about ten percent of my calories for my after dinner snack. Keeping meals about the same calories helps me keep track of how I trend for the day. I ask questions like, "If it is after lunch and I have twelve hundred calories left for the day, am I over or under?" If you end after lunch with about the same amount each day, then the question is easy to answer.

Exceptions will happen and life is good at throwing challenges at us. Maybe there was an unexpected pizza party in the middle of the day, or dinner gets delayed due to a late evening at work. But without going in with a plan, there can be no hope in ever meeting it. The more I made that plan a repeating habit, the more it happened without thinking about it.

Chapter 4: Starting Techniques

"If you want to make enemies, try to change something." - Woodrow Wilson

4.1. Calorie Density

Pizza, beef stew, hamburgers, and deep fried fish read like my dinner menu for a week. Every one of them was good and something I ate regularly. As I started my food journal, I looked at the calories between them. I was full for far fewer calories on beef stew than any of the others in that list. But I had beef stew every month or two. While the other foods, like pizza, I had multiple times within a week. Calories are about an average. Thus, I changed the frequency of the rotation. I rotated in lower calories foods, like beef stew, more often the higher calorie ones. To start I used the foods I already liked eating. No matter how bad your eating, there is something fewer calories than everything else, even if by a little bit. Furthermore, I still enjoyed pizza and deep fried fish, but every other week instead of week.

French fries went with each of those dinner choices. Meanwhile, mashed potatoes, another favorite, worked too. But, it took cartons of french fries to equal the fullness I get from one mound of mashed potatoes. Thus, I rotated the sides too. I had mashed potatoes and other lower calorie sides more than the higher calorie ones. As with the pizza, I still ate french fries but did not have them as often.

For desserts, I ate items like ice cream, cookies, and buttered popcorn. I could eat a whole carton of ice cream for thousands of calories and never feel content. But for two hundred calories I ate a giant bowl of buttered popcorn. Today, I use my air popper more than my ice cream scooper.

In the beginning, I did not know which foods would leave me feeling the most content for the least amount of calories. When I ate something, I began to pay attention to how I felt after eating it. I was not sure if the key was carbs, protein, fat, or some other mystical factor. As the meals built up, the answer became clear. The key to fullness was to pay attention to the calorie density of the food. To calculate take calories and divide by the weight in grams and times a hundred. That leaves me with calories per one hundred grams. Deep fried french fries are around three hundred calories per hundred grams, but the mashed potatoes I made tonight are eighty two calories per hundred grams. The better calorie bargain foods are like mashed potatoes, at or below hundred calories per hundred grams. In the early days, when the change was still new, I looked forward to dinners that hit the hundred mark. It meant I could eat in quantities like the old days and still be in my calorie goal.

The lower calorie choices offered other benefits. On the days with deep fried french fries and deep fried fish, I was tempted to keep eating, right up and beyond the calories need to maintain my weight. Yet, on the days of beef stew and mashed potatoes, I felt less compelled to keep eating. The lower calorie density food left me wanting more. It was like eating was more about how much weight of food you ate instead of the calories.

In addition, not only did I save calories, but I saved money. A bag of dehydrated beef stew was a third of the cost of a frozen pizza and feed the whole family. Meanwhile, air popped popcorn was cheaper than bird seed.

Why not eradicate all high calorie foods? The thought crossed my mind. My calorie success is a weekly average. As long as I average below the calories need to maintain my current weight, I will lose weight. Thus, I did not need to remove the high calorie foods. I was used to those foods, and it is a big step to let go of them. In time, I discovered I did not need to let go. Instead, I learned how to make them better for fewer calories. But, I did not want to upend everything I ate early on. I was trying to make a lifestyle change not make a round-trip to skinny and back as quick as possible.

When I did not plan the week ahead, I ended up with pizza and deep fried fish for dinner. I maintained my food journal in my mobile app, but it is not easy to look at what I have been eating for dinner across the last month. For that, I keep a wall calendar. Along with the dentist appointment, goes a note on what was for dinner last night. At a glance, I can see what I have been eating for dinner over the last month. At the start of each week, I use that to plan the upcoming week of dinners. I have two goals in planning. First, I make sure I do not neglect favorites, like pizza. Second, I ensure a good balance of lower calorie choices during the week. I do not want to be eating pizza today and then eat deep fried fish tomorrow. Something with a lower calorie density, like beef stew, will go between them.

If I ever longed for a high calorie favorite, the calendar gave me an objective view of how long it had been. Some weeks, I would be thinking it feels like I have not had pizza in months. Then the calorie would show I had it last Monday. That helped the craving go away. It felt ridiculous to pine over a food I ate the prior week. However, a large sausage and pepperoni pizza can at times stand up to any amount of ridiculousness. On those weeks, I planned it into the upcoming week. Having it once a week is better than every day in the week. Even every third day is better each day.

Beyond the first six months, I noticed my tastes changed. Ice cream remained a favorite. But, I hung out with other snacks for fewer calories. Every time I ate a mixing bowl's worth of buttered popcorn for two hundred calories, my fondness of popcorn grew. At the start, if I had to choose between giving up ice cream or popcorn, then I would have picked popcorn. But now, that would be reversed.

Moreover, the nature of a favorite changes. I used to want pizza every day. Pizza is still a favorite, but I get sick of pizza if I have it more than twice in a week. As my tastes got better, my calendar and planning also became about not getting sick of foods that I like. I used to plan to space out pizza to avoid the calories. Now I do it so that I do not get sick of pizza.

I learned how to make the original favorites come in better on calories. I used to eat two hamburgers for dinner and still do. Earlier on, I could not fit into two hamburgers to my dinner goal without breaking my goal. I felt cheated every time I had one hamburger for dinner. That motivated me to engineer the calories down using techniques I discuss later on. Today, I ate two hamburgers for dinner with enough left over for a snack. Thus, the higher calorie foods may not stay as high calorie if focus on engineering them to suite you.

4.2. Homemade Food

A box of cake mix comes off as offering very little choice. The box prescribes step by step what and how it should be prepared. But once you quit thinking about the given instructions, then that same box presents a world of calorie choices. I can leverage oil, butter, or applesauce. Likewise, I can make one giant pan or a dozen cup cakes. Not to mention the topping options. When I order a piece of cake at a restaurant, I do not have choices. A giant slice comes with the highest calorie choice for filling and icing. The only control I have is how much to eat, and I do not have a good history with that control. I am lucky to walk away for anything less than a full meal's worth of calories from that one piece of cake from the restaurant.

When I make lasagna at home, I load up it up with carrots, onions, and tomatoes. I use ground turkey and found six ounces of cheese plenty for a big tray. With the calories savings, I can afford to have bread with it. At a restaurant, the same side piece of bread would come soaked in butter and be more calories than the lasagna.

I was dining out at least once a week for dinner. I recognized the above early on and set on dining out less often. Like the higher calorie density foods, I rotate out the experience less often. Overtime, I went less because I asked myself "Why was I dining or ordering out as often as I was?" I realized it was not because the food was better.

I dined out because I wanted to eat without delay. However, it took time to drive there, wait to be seated, look over the menu, order the food, and wait for it to be cooked. It would be at least an hour in by the time I was eating. Worse, it took so long to eat, that I went on to over eat to make up for the time. I realized I could have cooked a meal before I had ordered the food. Even a drive-thru does not offer a big time savings. It takes at least twenty minutes for a round trip to a drive-thru. In that time, I could cook a hamburger, even if I started from a frozen patty. Thus, I ensured home cooking was quicker and easier.

For pizza, I cook the sausage topping, shred the cheese, and season the tomato sauce. This all goes into the fridge. When I get home from work, I assemble the pizza in a few minutes and then put into the oven. Using this method I can I have a more complex meal on the weekdays.

I did not use to plan; I dined out. As I started to plan, I began to use the slow cooker. I prepared all the ingredients the night before and stashed them in the fridge. In the morning, I dumped it into the slow cooker. Since I had brought together the ingredients the night before, I did not have to spend any morning time. When I get home from work, I have a home cooked meal waiting. There are other kitchen gadgets that save time. For instance, a pressure cooker can turn hours of cooking into minutes of cooking.

I cook a pound of breakfast sausage at a time. Then I freeze it and microwave pieces when I want some. On a weekday morning, I can have home cooked breakfast sausage in fifty seconds.

The key to success of using vegetables in cooking is to have them available to use. I peeled and diced onions, carrots, and other ingredients I wanted to use. Even for dry beans, I boiled a large batch and freeze so I can use them through the week. The freezer used to be where I put frozen pizza, but now it is where my meal starters live.

The best plans will not stop life from throwing surprises. I keep a few prepared entrées in my freezer and pantry, including a few processed choices. They are not what I reach for when I can avoid it. But, they are my last resort. I have another choice than the drive-thru.

Cooking was a hobby. Granted I was making unhealthy foods, but still it was a hobby. They say, "Never trust a skinny chef." I wondered how I would reconcile enjoying cooking with engineering calories? But, when I went to make something I discovered a different question. How do I balance optimizing my enjoyment and the calories?

Instead of a conflict, it was a new problem to solve and I love solving problems. Even though I had been cooking for years, it felt like something new had been added to my life. Today when I read a recipe, how to optimize the calories leaps to my mind as I read each line. Food is an integral part of life, and nothing brings it under your control better than making it a hobby.

When I was obese, I cooked for fun, when it fit my schedule. If I did not have the energy, I dined out. But, now I cook to balance both my health and enjoyment. What seemed like opposites turned into partners. Moreover, as I lost weight, I gained more energy. Now I have a mini-Thanksgiving dinner twice a month. As with the rest of the program, success builds more success.

4.3. Add-Ins

My homemade chili was a mix of tomato sauce, peppers, onions, beans, and spices. I took pride in growing my own peppers to use. Yet, I looked down at my bowl. I ate chili soaked crackers in a bed of cheese. I would have been better off buying chili cheese flavored crackers. Many of the add-ins I was using were becoming the entrée. They dominated the taste, texture, and calories. The crackers and cheese in the chili bowl were more than double the calories of the chili. I asked myself "What did I set out to eat?" The crackers, cheese, and other add-ins are there to accent the food, not replace it. They are like salt and pepper. Good in small amounts, terrible in large. Of course, I had to figure out how to make that transition.

The first technique was separating the add-in from the food. I used to crumble up the crackers and stir them into my chili like I was mixing cake batter. Now I keep the crackers on the side in a separate plate. I dip each one into the bowl of chili. I have a crunchy cracker with chili on top instead of a mushy cracker waded in chili. I discovered an added benefit. When I do that, both the crackers and the chili taste better.

My second technique was to ask "How much of the add-in I need?" This was best seen on my hamburgers. My hamburger had so many calorie add-ins I would not have noticed if I had left out the actual hamburger patty. I started with the mayo, which was the highest calorie add-on. The serving size, listed on the nutrition panel, was a tablespoon. Yet, an ice cream scooper would have been a better measuring tool for the amounts of mayo I used. I took the smaller serving size as a suggestion and tried to work down to that amount. At first, I went to three servings of mayo per hamburger, but over time I worked down to one serving. Moreover, the mayo felt right at that amount. It provided a good accent to the meat and did not over power it, as it had been doing. Plus I started saving money. I bought a jar of mayo every week. Now, I go a month or more without buying any.

As I looked at the hamburger, I realized the hamburger bun was an add-on in a way. Over time, I trended up to larger and larger hamburger buns. The bun over hung the meat patty by inches. I started downsizing my buns until they were the same size as the meat patty. As a side benefit, this let me use less mayo.

Third, I reasoned with myself. I make pulled pork once a month. I smoke a pork butt for twelve hours. The meat turns out tender enough that it falls apart at the touch. Every piece of meat tasted like the hard wood it was smoked in. It was worth its weight in calories, which is better than gold. It will forever be in my favorite food list. However, I used to take the meat and dump a jar of two dollar BBQ sauce on it. Enough that BBQ sauce would fall off the sandwich and over the plate. Once I started paying attention to calories, I asked "What is the point of smoking for twelve hours?" I could have made it in the oven or slow cooker and still dumped cheap BBQ sauce on it. I defeated the work I put into making it. When I thought of it that way, it was like getting punched in the stomach. I scaled back the BBQ sauce. Sometimes I do not even use BBQ sauce. I want to taste every second of that twelve hour smoke period.

The worst add-ins began with a high calorie food. Take deep fried french fries. Restaurants offer these "loaded" by adding on bacon and cheese. The add-ins dwarf even the deep frying process. In desserts, my favorite was ice cream. But it did not feel complete unless I added fudge, nuts, sprinkles, pieces of candy bar. I needed fifty forms of sugar in one bowl. High calorie items can fit in a food plan. But, it becomes difficult to work in high calorie items with high calorie add-ins. If I want to splurge on something high calorie, then I want to enjoy what I am setting out to splurge on, not fifty other things I put on top of it.

I did not realize I was super sizing my calories with the add-ins. It took keeping the food journal and examining the calorie breakdown. Before then, I lived in fat bliss.

I started to think all add-ins were dangerous, but it turned out to be the ones I ate the most. Some add-ins were so low that it made sense to eat more of them. For instance, I "loaded" my hamburger with lettuce, peppers, onions, and tomato. These add-ins contributed flavor notes, helped leave me fuller, and were less than twenty calories all together. I stack in as many of them as I can. Now I eat peppers on my hamburger, like I used to eat mayo on my hamburger.

Meanwhile, I discovered a middle ground. For instance, ketchup is twenty calories per serving, and one serving is enough for a hamburger or two. When I try to use two or three servings of ketchup on a single hamburger, the extra serving amount falls off the bun onto the plate. Even if I dip the hamburger in it as I eat, three servings are still under a hundred calories. Thus, it has some calories, but is tough to overeat. For those add-ins, I added them in moderation, but did not feel I had to be as cautious.

4.4. Why Do I Eat?

I did not have a good answer to an important question. Why do I eat? The answer was never apparent. It was not because I was hungry. During my weight loss, I returned to that question as often as the question of how to lower calories.

I solved a tough problem at work - deep dish pizza. It is Friday - fried chicken. A new Walking Dead episode is premiering tonight - buffet. Plus, there is a birthday or holiday around the corner that requires food to celebrate. Even if it is one month out, the time to celebrate is now. I did not realize how much I was celebrating with food until my wife pointed it out. Sometimes it takes someone outside of us to let us know what we are doing.

I found other ways to celebrate. My current weekend celebration is a family trip to places like the zoo or museum. Something that gets me up and about. I am trying to explore other ways to enjoy life. I even found a low calorie food celebration in a trip to the local apple orchard. It is near impossible to overeat apples. I say that after finding five apples was the maximum I could eat in a single setting even when I was obese. Now that I am much less, I get sick of them after two. Thus, I do not mind a lower calorie apple orchard celebration.

I kept other food celebrations, but engineered the calories to levels that fit in my plan. Gone are the days where my food celebration was a ten thousand calorie buffet trip. I celebrate the new episode of Walking Dead with buttered popcorn. That is now a Sunday tradition for my wife and me. For my birthday, we used to get a cake with enough for servings for sixty four skinny people. Instead, my wife makes homemade cupcakes. I can eat one or two without going over my calorie goals. Plus, homemade cupcakes with "Happy Birthday Daddy" written on them made by your family mean more than any cake that can ever be bought.

I kept a bag of candy sitting on the counter. As I walked by, I grabbed a few pieces. Once they were gone, I returned to grab a few more. One of the first changes I made was to remove the bag of candy from the counter. I put it on top of the fridge, in the far back, in a box. There was no chance of walking by and engaging in impulse eating. I had to think I wanted candy and then hunt it down. I ate less candy without having to think about it.

The same technique worked for high calorie desserts and meals. I used to keep my brownies on the counter, but now I freeze them after baking. I put them behind the frozen broccoli, which is to fat people like garlic to vampires. Storing in the fridge does not work as well because I am always opening it. Brownies in the fridge are ones I will eat later in the day. Brownies in the freezer are for another day. That is my new motto.

When I walked into a movie theater, the aroma of butter hit me and eating popcorn came to mind. It was a conditioned habit but changeable. I ate popcorn at home before going to remove the temptation. Plus, after a few times of not getting popcorn at the movies the urge fades, as I get a new habit of not buying popcorn.

At work, people bring in treats in the morning and sit them in the break room. I went to the break room and ate a bagel or two with extra walnut cream cheese. Yet, I continued to have a normal sized lunch at the normal time. But then I realized that bagels do not age well during the day. An eight am bagel is like a candy bar, but a one pm bagel is like a rock. Thus, I quit going to the break room during the prime time. When I go by later, I remind myself that it is a one pm bagel as I go by.

In the day time, I ate a sizable meal every five hours. Once the night hit, my meal clock kept running. As I stayed up late past my normal bed time, I craved another meal. When I started, it was tough to get to sleep. I would wake in the middle of the night. Eating seemed like an easy way to help. As I lost weight, it became easier to go to sleep. Then one day I woke up without having a midnight snack because it was the right time to wake up. Good sleeping habits help that night time temptation.

Other times I ate more because it felt like a value. I could super size my meal for a dollar. But it was an attempt for them to save on garbage costs, which is where the extra food deserved to be. If I feel content with the regular size portion, then why do I need more? By the time I factored in feeling sick from overeating, not sleeping well, and long term health costs, the super size option was not a bargain.

4.5. Inner Toddler

The modern toddler evolved to subsist on chicken nuggets, with a fish stick added on the weekend for variety. No matter how much I insisted my children eat, they continued to see the food in front of them as optional. Though, I will have to be careful because one day they will cross that chicken nugget phase. My childhood lesson lived on with me long after crossing my phase. I have lost track of how many times in my adult life I ate something I did not like because I felt I should not waste it. I would rather gorge myself on a cake about to go bad, rather than throw it out. Food put in front of me feels like an obligation I have to uphold. For me, it was anything but optional, which is why my children are confusing. I never knew there was a choice.

Should I be treating food as an obligation? I gave into my inner toddler. Food on the floor is more interesting than food in the mouth. If I do not want it or it does not taste good, I do not eat. I am not afraid to spit out food. At the grocery store on sample day, my wife laughs at how many samples I spit out. From the taste, I understand why they are giving away the food. One day I may even learn to quit taking the sample when offered.

The grocery store had a new extra large cake. For two or more days, I gorged on it between candy bars, but half remained in the fridge. The one solution that came to mind was to keep eating it. The thought of throwing it away seemed like lighting cash on fire. I asked "What would my inner toddler do?" My hands shook as I carried the cake over to the garbage can. I paused for a length of time that seemed long enough to bake a cake. Yet, I held tight. It felt like I was in a movie standing over a volcano with a sacrifice I held dear. Then I let go. It dropped into the garbage in an instant. I breathed out, for the first time since taking it out of the fridge. But as I stared at it down in the trash, I knew I did the right thing and I felt power. Power over cake - I have never seen that one as a movie super power, but it should be.

From that day forward, I never bought a cake that size again. If I had not thrown it out, I would have bought the same size again. Not only that, I would have bought the double extra large size when it hit the shelf. Every future trip I would tell myself, I ate the smaller size last time. But now every time I saw the extra large size, I remembered my sacrifice to the volcano. When was the last time you bought a smaller size because the larger size went to waste?

I thought over the way I like to cook things. I have been trying to develop more picky tastes. French fries need to be sliced and seasoned a certain way. You know, the right way. Anything less than the right way is junk not worth eating. I like it the way I like, and I am not going to make due with anything less. If that sounds ambiguous and subjective, then it should. That way it leaves me the most flexibility to embrace my inner toddler.

The last thing I learned from my toddler was to stop eating when you are done. If I got him to eat something, there was a point where he quit eating. He says "I'm done" and wants to go play. This amount of food had nothing to do with how much food had been placed on his plate.

Chapter 5: Substitution Techniques

"He who is not courageous enough to take risks will accomplish nothing in life." - Muhammad Ali

5.1. Different Varieties

On the grocery store shelf, bottles of barbecue sauce stood with pictures of firewood or bees. They had names like hardwood fire and honey sweet. I picked up bottles to compare. I considered how it might taste on my pulled pork sandwich. The picture, name, flavor description, and price drove my decision. But, I never gave thought to the calories. When I did, I saw flavors like honey sweet varied by a hundred calories between brands. Meanwhile, flavors like hardwood fire were twenty five calories per serving. I asked myself if I could identify with hardwood fire.

I used to eat enough ice cream to feed a small village. My main factor on ice cream selection was how much candy, chocolate, nuts, or caramel was added. When I was in a healthy mood, I purchased frozen yogurt or sugar-free ice cream with the same add-ins. Once I compared calories, I discovered some of my healthier ice cream choices were higher in calories. The add-ins I was going after would make frozen seaweed high in calories. I asked myself if I could be happy with only candy or caramel added and not both.

Hamburgers had been in at least one meal every month of my life. Yet, in the recent years, the bun took over. It provided more space than any meat patty could ever dream of needing. The buns were over three hundred calories each. Next to them was a bun that was one and half times the size of the meat patty. I asked myself if that size would work for me.

Each of my prior examples saved a hundred calories per serving. I used to compare with price and taste, but the grocery store shelves had a new light once I added calories as a factor. I ate the same kinds of foods, but tried new flavors and brands. As a side benefit, I ate more variety. This technique is as simple as it sounds. It was foundational because I learned to be analytical about the calories in food.

There are potential missteps. My first thought at finding lower calorie versions was that I could eat more. If I wanted to stay obese, then that would have been fine. But I wanted to create a calorie deficit. Thus, I kept eating the same amount. I did not step down amounts until months later. If I ate the same foods in the same amounts, but each had fewer calories, then I have created my calorie deficit.

There are items labeled healthy, natural, organic, and ancient. Some of the labels are misleading, with all organic having non-organic ingredients, or chemical flavoring used for the natural label. They are like the product picture, a false image used for marketing. I skip past the mountain picture and inner Zen names and look for the calories.

I was comparing ice cream. One brand was ten calories less for a half cup than another brand. Both were the same flavor. I put the lower calorie one in my cart. But, it did not have less add-ins, so I was not sure how it was fewer calories. Then I noticed that the serving size in grams was different between the two of them. They both said half a cup, but had a different number of grams. When I divided out the calories per gram, they were the same amount of calories. For food like ice cream, weight is the more important measure. For potato chips, maybe the number of chips might be better. I learned to compare like serving sizes.

Most of the calorie difference between two foods is from sugar. As the name hints, this is true for hardwood fire and honey sweet BBQ sauce. But for items like apple juice I was confused. Next to the bottle I was buying, there was one labeled half the calories. How can any type of apple juice be half the calories of another? Did they invent a new type of apple? The nutrition panel showed everything, from calories through vitamin C, as being halved. This implied filler with no calories had diluted the juice - water. Moreover, the ingredient list hinted at more water added. I already dilute juice with more water, so the lower calorie apple juice did not offer any benefit. It would have been a worse option because it was priced the same.

Meanwhile, I compared chicken breast. One package was ninety calories per ounce. Another was one hundred ten calories per ounce. Before I bought the lower calorie one, I wondered how can two different packages of chicken breast be different calories? If it was breaded, then I could have understood. In theory, the diet and type of chicken could influence the calories. But like the apple juice that was not it. As I examined the packages, I saw how they did it. The label reported "injected with a flavor enhancing fluid." Removing the marketing gimmick, that meant water. It added weight, but no calories. Thus, the lower calorie chicken breast was diluted with more water. I bought the kind with less water added. I planned to use less chicken breast in my recipe. Then when I went to use it, I felt cheated using fifteen ounces of chicken breast instead of a full pound. No matter how much I reminded myself that it was water weight. I ended up having to add the missing ounce which canceled out the calorie and cost savings. The second time I bought the lower calorie chicken breast. It may be diluted with water. But, if I cannot bring myself to use less of it, then I am better off with the watered-down version. I found this truer in the early days. Once your healthy weight, everything is possible, but you have got to get past those obese pounds first.

Beyond those foods are other processed foods, like mayo. There are many different ways to make all of them for fewer calories. When it is not apparent like sugar difference, I do not know if they are adding water or cheap filler. I decided it did not matter because higher calorie food has cheap filler added. It is called sugar. I can learn to use an ounce less of chicken breast. But, I do not know how to dilute mayo or use less of it below a certain point.

5.2. Light Versions

I eyed the mayo bottles on the shelf. The lids were blue, red, orange, yellow, and every shade in between. A light sea blue colored lid stood out. It felt light in my hand, despite being the same size package as regular. It was a light mayo variety. I had many questions. What would this taste like? Was it less healthy than the regular? Is it worth it? It was only a few dollars, yet I paused as if I was buying a car. I was trying the lower calorie versions of everything, but until that point, I had not ventured into "light" varieties. Still, the light mayo was thirty five calories, which was half of the regular. Two servings was enough difference to be half way to a serving of ice cream. I dived into the light sea blue. I approached the first hamburger like a kid being told they are eating peas for dinner. But as I ate, it dawned on me. I tasted no difference.

After light mayo, I tried light buttermilk ranch dressing. It came in at half the calories too. I tasted a minor difference. The difference was like that between two brands. It still came across with the notes of buttermilk ranch, and it pepped up the salad at the same. Most of the light foods are like mayo, no noticeable difference, but a few are like the dressing, with a slight difference.

Most of the time, the lighter calorie choices are the same price as the regular. This is true of both salad dressing and mayo. But it is not true of all foods. When I went looking for lighter sliced cheese, I found two light options. One was thirty calories per slice. It was about the same price as regular with a few less slices per package. Next to it, there was another brand that offered a twenty five calorie per slice choice. It was two dollars more per pack. Five calories was not worth two dollars. It takes ten slices before I am at fifty calories.

I spent premium dollars to use premium maple syrup. However, one bottle lasted long enough for the next grocery store trip. I looked at the regular pancake syrup choices. Some were made of pure corn syrup and more calories than maple syrup. I avoided those. I found one with less, then worked down into light pancake syrup. There was a sugar free package syrup for a tenth of the calories of maple syrup. I could pour it on like water, but it tasted like water. Thus, I stopped at the light pancake syrup. You will not like everything and do not always have to pursue the lowest calorie choice. But there is value in exploring. You never learn any other way.

Reduced fat and fat-free mayo jars were sitting right among the others. These are marketing gimmick choices. They are not lower calories. They add more sugar and salt to help make up for the lower fat. However, I have never eaten a high fat item and walked away hungry. Moreover, many forms of fat, like that in olive oil and peanut butter, are good for you.

The one exception on fat is dairy products, like milk and cheese. The amount of fat is the reason dairy products have different calories. As milk flows, they separate out the fat. Then depending on what they are making, they add back in a set amount of fat. Two percent milk and whole milk come out of the same cow utter line. One has more milk fat added back into it. Cheese made from whole milk, 2% milk fat, or skim milk will say less fat and will be lower in calories. But other than dairy, I do not use level of fat as a proxy for calorie comparison.

The skinny me told me to merge the sections on different varieties and light varieties into one section. But I remembered back to my fat self. Light varieties were something different onto themselves. I do not understand why, but I had some built-in aversion to light foods. A light label implied healthy, skinny, and everything I was not. Wade into the light varieties and do not rush. Light mayo was my gateway light food. I spent a few weeks getting used to seeing light food containers in the pantry before I branched out into the other light foods.

5.3. Similar but Different

When I was I fat, I used ground beef in tacos, chili, and beef stew. When I ate chicken for dinner, I ate beef for lunch. If I could have made hot dogs and potato chips from ground beef, then I would have. But, ground beef packs the calories. I tried comparing ground sirloin, ground round, and the other lean ratings. As the calories went down, the cost of ground beef went up to steak prices. Across from the ground beef was ground turkey. It was less than two thirds the calories and the price. I pictured chili and tacos crossed with a thanksgiving dinner and could see myself throwing out the food. But, I pushed through the image. Two thirds the calories was too tempting. The first dish I tried it in was chili. With the beans, peppers, and seasoning, it stood the best chance. I finished after eating three bowls of chili and remembered that I had substituted ground turkey. After that, I made tacos with it. Now when I see ground beef on a recipe, I read it as ground turkey.

After a few months, I looked for more calories savings and wondered if I could beat ground turkey. I used beans for half of the ground turkey. Beans are traditional in tacos and chili. For non-traditional dishes, like spaghetti, I ran the cooked beans through the blender with some water or tomato sauce. People, who claim they hate beans, ask for seconds. Beans are cheap, low calorie, and a good protein source. Plus, they added another flavor tone to the dish. It was not like I was making due with a sub-par food, but rather enhancing the dish with a new flavor.

Months into that, I wondered if I could beat beans. I asked, "What goes with beans?" Rice came to mind. This does not offer protein, but I was only replacing half the ground turkey, not all of it. Plus, my food journal showed I swam in protein, so I was not concerned. It gave me another option for both calories and flavor. I would not have been able to replace even an ounce of meat with rice at the start, but the months of experience on other items opened up the possibility.

With the amount of ice cream I was eating, I knew I needed a substitute. There were other flavors and brands. But, for the amount I wanted to eat, it still was not enough. I branched out into close cousins of ice cream. I explored frozen yogurt and sherbet. They offered savings, but not to the degree I needed. I found the best calories savings for a frozen treat were fruit popsicles. They are like eating summer on a stick, but do not offer that dairy feel. It was nice to have another frozen treat to rotate on the calories, but it was not a replacement. Meanwhile, I taste tested many Greek yogurt flavors in pursuit of one I liked. Then one day, I took plain vanilla greek yogurt and mixed in frozen blueberries. It was like discovering a new flavor of candy bar. Better yet, it was something I could eat in a big ice cream bowl without spending ice cream level calories. I would never mistake the taste for ice cream. But the dairy, texture, and frozen fruit trick my primal mind into thinking it is a type of ice cream. Today, I eat Greek yogurt with frozen fruit as part of breakfast, and the ice cream cravings have gone with the pounds.

Substituting similar but different foods was the largest contributor to my calorie deficit. If I had known the flavors I was missing out on, I would have done it for taste alone. There are a number of places to get suggestions for substitutions to try. Look in the grocery store for items placed near each other, like ground turkey and ground beef. Or, foods that have the same ingredient, like dairy in ice cream and yogurt. Or, foods that are paired together often, like meat and beans. Explore.

5.4. Will Work for Calories

Similar but different wins often, but there are times I cannot accept a substitute. In high school health class, there was an assignment to keep a food journal for a week. Mine said hamburger for lunch and dinner for the every entry of the week. My love of hamburgers is the one place were ground turkey failed me. It did not taste bad as a turkey burger, but different. I tried bean based burgers too. They showed me new spices and flavors. My menu grew with new food options that tasted good and were low calorie. My average calorie goals were improved. But, eating a turkey or bean burger left me wanting a beef burger. They were different songs in the same concert. But nothing less than a beef hamburger would do. It was at the top of my engineering list, and I peered into the center of it.

Store bought ground beef is about three hundred calories per four ounces. At first, I was desperate for a calorie efficient hamburger. I bought the leanest beef I could, sparing no expense because I could have bought steak for the price. Worse, it came out dry as rubber. The turkey and bean burgers beat that one. Then I looked wider in the grocery aisle. Not too far over were packs of chuck roast. They were close to the same price and were a fraction of the calories at two hundred calories per four ounces. I was confused on how it could be fewer calories. The ground beef at the store was labeled ground chuck. They must put extra fat or reject meat into it. I shuddered at the thought remembering how many hamburgers past I have eaten from store ground beef. Next, I needed an easy way to turn ground chuck into hamburgers because if it was not easy I would not do it.

I have a meat grinder attachment for my mixer. It is an expedition to find and put together the pieces. The beef has to be cut into one inch cubes. If a bigger piece slips in, then it clogs up the feed tube. Afterward, it as much fun to wash as scrubbing the floor. My love of hamburgers might have been enough to endure that, but first I researched for an easier way.

The food processor works fine. Cut off a piece of roast and hit go. Within a minute, it is ground as well as store bought. If you want to get fancy, experiment with course grinds, but it is fine if you do not want to mess with it. The only problem I had was not to overload with too much meat at once. I found about a pound at a time works well in mine. My starting goal was to reduce the calories, but I found more. My wife does not share my enthusiasm for hamburgers, but she asks for these. The weight loss was nice, but finding the perfect hamburger made the journey worth it on its own.

Grinding a chuck roast every time I wanted a hamburger would involve too much washing of the food processor for my tastes. When chuck roast goes on sale, I buy five pounds of it and work through it in small batches. I pat it out into hamburger patties and freeze. Then when I want a hamburger, I take from freezer to pan - no thawing needed. Frozen hamburger patties from the grocery store rate with drive-thru hamburgers, but the freeze does not alter the home ground ones.

A hamburger was nice, but a cheeseburger was the ice cream with fudge drops. However, the slice of cheese I was adding was a third of the calories of the hamburger patty. Plus, slice cheese came packaged in defined whole slices. Trying to use a slice and a half divided between two hamburgers leaves me hating the cheese. Not to mention the slice cheese tastes like a cheese product, not cheese.

First, I found a sharp cheddar slice cheese made from skim milk. This was half the calories of regular American sliced cheese. The cheddar flavor was better than the American processed flavor. But the original was a cheese product, and this was too. I wondered if I could improve both calories and taste.

A block cheddar cheese made from two percent milk wins the cheese taste contest. I spent a minute running a block of cheddar cheese over a cheese grater. A half ounce more than replaces a single slice of cheese. It has the same calories as the sliced skim milk cheese. I used to do the math to calculate out an exact number of calories. Now I do simple math and divide into half or quarter ounce. The extra calories I saved with three sixteenths of an ounce are not worth my time.

I never looked at the calories in pre-shredded cheese, as I hate the taste of the wax they coat it in to extend the shelf life. Home shredded cheese lasts for about a week in the fridge in an air tight container. It freezes well too. Though at my house, an eight ounce blocks does not live a week.

For dinner, I eat two cheeseburgers. At first, it was like eating pizza for dinner in terms of calorie impact. The earlier techniques helped with the mayo and bun. But discovering I could do work to gain calories on the beef and cheese was like finding an oil well in the backyard. The calories went down enough to allow me to add more in and upgrade the bun to a homemade sourdough bun. The bun in itself makes the sandwich. I also have enough calories left after dinner for my post dinner snack.

The food processor works for chicken breast too. I do not do that to save calories, as ground chicken breast is low calories, but I save dollars. Whole chicken breast is cheap, but ground chicken breast is as expensive as lean ground beef. Thus, I buy a few pounds of cheap chicken breast and freeze some ground chicken breast to use in recipes. I would do the same for turkey if I could get raw turkey cheap enough.

There is one risk in this. I have to make sure I measure out the amount. I am never tempted to measure out more hamburger meat for a patty because I am making and freezing pounds of patties in advance. However, there was a temptation to lay on a few more grams of shredded cheese. A few more are not worth the thought either way, but the danger is that a few could turn into double or more. Thus, if you keep overeating the shredded cheese, then go back to the slice cheese. The plastic wrapping forces you into a serving size.

If someone would have told me I could have eaten better and saved calories at the same time for a small bit of work, I would have never believed them. This method is not as applicable to all food categories as the prior techniques, but it wins when it is applicable. Moreover, it appeals to my whole food preferences, since I start with minimally processed ingredients. On the contrary, the grocery store hamburger patties, processed cheese slices, and other things are showcases of modern chemistry.

5.5. One Step More

Hamburger success left me wondering what else could I trade time for calories, even if it involved over one step. I tried pork sausage next. A trip through the food processor grinds it up and incorporates spices at the same time. Every month, I buy a pork butt to smoke into pulled pork. I bought a pound or two larger and cut off the extra to use for sausage making. Sometimes pork butt is sold as country pork chops. You could use that too. The difference between Italian, breakfast, and other sausages is in the added spices. I have not made standard breakfast sausage yet. Every time I start, I find another seasoning mix that interests me. Johnny Earles's Spicy Sausage recipe has been on my morning breakfast plate recently. Even better is I cannot buy that flavor at the grocery store.

Home ground pork sausage rivals hamburger meat in calorie savings. Pork butt is loaded with enough fat I can smoke a whole roast for over twelve hours. Afterward, it comes out as a tender as butter. Yet, pork butt clocks in at two hundred twenty calories per four ounces. Meanwhile, store bought sausage is three hundred fifty calories per four ounces. I assume they add straight fat or worse into it. I do not want to know though because I used to eat it.

When I ate breakfast, I needed something I could make while still drowsy. Store bought cereal was there for me. I ate it every morning. The stuff is like a drug. No sooner than I finished one hit, I was hungry for more. I debated if I should skip breakfast and eat a bigger lunch. Yet, when I ate sausage, oatmeal, or pancakes for breakfast I could ride to lunch without questioning the value of breakfast. I needed something different but still quick. Nothing beats the "dump in a bowl and go" speed preparation of cereal. Thus, I checked if I could make my own cereal and found homemade granola recipes. It requires a few more steps to make ahead of time than the earlier examples but not by much. It assemblies into one mixing bowl and is dumped onto one cookie tray for baking. I spend less than ten minutes making a batch of granola that lasts for two weeks. The grocery store cereal was so high calorie, it was not hard to beat. This gave me room to add in real pecans and honey and still come under. As I will say many times, I am not out for zero calories. I am here to eat filling food that is worth the calories it has. My granola does not come with the same farm pictures as store bought but deserves it more.

I make spice blends for tacos, chili, and spaghetti. This saves me over a hundred calories. And like the pork sausage seasoning mixes, I gain new options I cannot buy. All of which taste better than the packet that has a sell by date over a year out. While spice jars can be pricey, they last months or longer. In the long run, I come out cheaper than buying the seasoning packets.

The further I went along, the more I asked, "What do I eat?" Then I would see what it took to make a homemade version of that and if the calorie and cost savings was worthwhile. Meanwhile, I could, but do not make mayo because I use little of it. If I knew this technique right at the start, I could have saved a bundle on mayo. But with the way my tastes have changed over time, mayo has become a lesser food in my life.

I advise going slow into this. Try one food at a time. Start with the one that is the dearest to you. Once making that one is a natural part of your routine, then consider if you want to branch into another. Do not feel you have to do this on every possible thing every single time you want it. I can make all this homemade food now because I have made each one often enough to make it in my sleep. Then after getting to that level of comfort, I added other items. For instance, homemade peanut butter, another easy one, is something I only started making in the last few months. When I make something new for the first few times, I have to pause, double check things, and learn what I am doing. But if you can do this, then you will save money and calories and eat food that is less processed and tastes better.

Chapter 6: Category Techniques

"Happiness is when what you think, what you say, and what you do are in harmony." - Mahatma Gandhi

6.1. Just Fruit

Many an obese night, I spent with a giant bowl overfilling with ice cream. I found better tasting substitutes that can overfill the bowl for a fraction of the calories. Last summer, I went through bowls of strawberries like I used to with ice cream. Yet, I spent a fraction of the calories. Watermelon was better. It cost trivial calories to gorge on watermelon until I was sick of it. Heaping bowls of fruit were of a different calorie magnitude than ice cream, candy bars, or cookies; but they tasted better and are healthier.

Not all fruit was as low calorie as strawberry and watermelon, so I did not eat overflowing bowls of every kind. As with anything else, I adjusted based on the calories. Know thy calories. Still, I sometimes got the urge for mountains of higher calorie fruit like bananas. I did not worry though. It took five bananas to start to counter a five hundred calorie deficit. I got sick of bananas after two, so I was safe. Apples were my go to bad boy fruit. If I felt like I needed to eat at the end of the day and did not care about how many calories I had left, I ate an apple. A whole apple is fifty calories. I felt rebellious, but the calories fit inside rounding error for the day.

When I ate something, I wanted to another something, whatever that something was, without pausing between. However, fruit had a built-in pause between pieces. I had to peel and chop up another apple or cut off the tops of more strawberries. Even if I was taking it out of the freezer and microwaving, there was a pause to microwave more. The pauses between slowed down my eating. From built-in pauses to lower calorie profiles, fruits are low risk sweets.

Where does eating fruit lead to? Eating more varieties of fruit. Even at a regular grocery store, there were many fruits I never tried or ate in the past. Take plantains. They are a cousin of the banana and sit on the shelf next to the bananas. In years past, I never noticed them, but I am sure they were not a recent import. They are healthy too. Most people think carrots when they think of vitamin A, but I think of plantains. I do not understand how I ever lived without eating some of my "newly discovered" fruits, such as plantains, pineapple, and others. I never ate any of these growing up, but they are on my shopping list now. If you pressed me in the past, I could have named a few fruits, but today I can name fruit after fruit I eat. In the past, I felt like there are no new foods out there, but with fruits, I keep discovering new. There are many fruits literally growing on trees, not to mention bushes. During the journey, my tastes sharpened. The different types of apples taste like different fruits to me. Before, I could only taste a difference in sweetness, but now I taste a range of flavor tones in each.

Bananas are sitting on my counter, apples in the refrigerator, strawberries in the freezer, and several cans of fruit in the cabinet. I decide what to get based on convenience, taste, and cost. I keep cans of mixed fruit cocktail on hand for the kids. During apple season, I keep a bowl of sliced apple in the fridge for the same reason. The taste and costs vary over the year. Fresh strawberries become dirt cheap and tasty when they are in season but are the opposite outside of that season. Thus, I buy frozen strawberries whenever they are outside of season. My goal is to have fruit on hand. In my kitchen, you will trip over at least three kinds of fruit before finding something dangerous to eat. Fruit is like calorie flood sandbags.

Fruit is cheap. I buy ten pounds of bananas for about the price of a single happy meal. Those ten pounds of bananas last my family for a week with a few left over to freeze for smoothies. Plus, there might be a sale on fruit. When I have freezer space to spare, I stock up on sales. At the end of summer, my freezer was loaded with strawberry, blackberry, and grapes. When fruit is in season I look for local farms or orchards that I can buy it from. I make regular trips to a local orchard in the summer. I do not pay extra for organic because I do not think it is worth it. Also, if you have a bit of yard space and are looking for a fun hobby, consider growing fruit. For instance, strawberries grow like weeds and will yield buckets of fruit from even a small planting.

I learned some bad habits as a child. I ate strawberries rolled around in table sugar. I do not know if it is better or worse to say I even added sugar to store bought cereal, which already has half a bag of sugar added. When I came back to eat fruit with a more calorie conscience view, the first thing I did was to quit adding sugar on fruit. If the fruit does not taste good without adding sugar, then something is wrong with the fruit.

Sometimes frozen fruit is frozen with added sugar. I avoid that and look for no sugar added on the label. But with canned fruit, it is canned in a liquid which may add calories. Water adds no calories, but is not always a choice. The various forms that canned fruit can take can be confusing. Rather than explain it, I will advise what I do. Look at the calorie label on the can and compare to the other ones sitting next to it on the shelf. You do not have to learn which level of sugar syrup has the same amount of calories as juice if you remember to read labels. Plus, reading labels helps you compare any two foods.

Fruit on its own is my main stay, but I like to mix it up. Fruit with one step more becomes a whole other treat. Take a banana. I can slice it and freeze. No need to dip in chocolate, frozen banana slices are a treat in themselves. I keep some ready in the top drawer of the freezer. My toddler asks for pieces when he sees the freezer open. Dehydrated pineapple is my sole reason for owning a dehydrator. Apple slices with cinnamon sprinkled on them are like a candy bar. Those do not require any cooking. However, if you are up for cooking, you gain even more options. I boil sweet apples down into applesauce. Starting with sweet apples removes the need to add any sugar. It is possible to get into more formal desserts, but my point is fruit with one step becomes a whole other treat. This is the one paragraph in the whole book that made me want to go eat what while I was writing about it. I get a pain when I type candy bar, but I think fireworks when I start typing what I can do with fruit.

6.2. Fruit Based Deserts

When I was obese, homemade candy bars were the pinnacle of my dessert cooking. I used regular sugar, powdered sugar, corn syrup, caramel, milk chocolate, and little else. It tasted like sugar was dancing the tango with sugar and more sugar was joining into the festival. A few other fellow fat people told me it was too rich for them. A single batch clocked in over five thousand calories. Looking back, I try not to remember how much of one batch I ate the first night I made them. That was the kind of dessert that helped me stay fat. Nothing more than forms of sugar dancing, no real substance.

The one fruit-based dessert I ate was apple pie. Even that was on a holiday and was loaded with more sugar than apples. But as I ate more fruit, I thought about fruit-based desserts. I made apple crisp, blueberry cobbler, and pudding berry cake. Fruit was playing center stage with sugar along for the ride. These were desserts with flavor substance and low on calories. I used to make cookies every week. Now I make one of those twice a week and v remember the last time I made cookies.

As I looked through my newer cookbooks, I saw pages with full color photos of an endless stream of cookie recipes but not any fruit desserts. In my older cookbooks, I found what I needed. Also, any online search will reveal other options. Sometimes I find things I would not have thought of. For instance, I found a good strawberry rugelach recipe in one of my older cookbooks. I did not even know what rugelach was; let alone how to make strawberries play center in it.

Before I make any fruit dessert recipe for the first time, I go over it and make tweaks. For instance, I came across an apple spice cake recipe. The spices sounded like they would taste good on their own, but other parts needed adjustments. First, I read cake in the recipe title, but planned to make it as cupcakes to help define the servings. In the past, I overate cake since serving size is subjective. But I did not overeat cupcakes, since their serving size is defined. Second, I used sweet apples instead of tart. Many fruit desserts call for tart fruit, then say to add two cups of sugar. If I like eating the fruit on its own, then I know I do not need as much sugar. Third, the recipe called for half an apple. That was an amount for "made with apple", but I wanted "made of apple." I increased the amount to five apples. When I make a fruit-based dessert, I aim to make fruit the main ingredient, not as a flavoring for sugar. That was a key misstep with most of the fruit dessert recipes you will find. Each recipe may require experimentation to find the right amount of fruit. But, each experiment is a delicious one. Last, I lowered down the sugar to a reasonable level. You will learn as you go how much you need, but it is not what is listed. It might be at first, but after a few months, it will not be. In the end, I had an apple-based cupcake that danced with cinnamon, nutmeg, cloves, and cocoa.

For fruit pies, like the prototypical apple pie, I try to minimize the breading or make something comparable. For instance, I eat more apple crisp instead of apple pie. With apple pie, there is a breading crust underneath the apple filing and on top. With apple crisp, there is granola on top and no calories from below the apples. I still make apple pie. But as with other higher calorie foods, I rotate in apple crisp more often. And when I make apple pie, I make sure it does not become a crust pie.

I mentioned how fruit with one more step adds variety. When you think of fruit-based desserts, this leads into simple one-step desserts that are nowhere as complex as apple pie. For instance, I cut up two hundred grams of plantains. Then, I fry them in a tablespoon each of honey and butter. The aroma is like honeybees are making honey from cinnamon. My toddler eats it and requests more. That is the best seal of food approval I know.

Disclaimer: You must be careful in adding sugar to fruit. I keep the sugar under control and plan in for the calories. Also, I do not lump fruit and sugar with regular fruit but treat it as a dessert. The way desserts were meant to be. I enjoy them and have them many nights of the week. But I still eat more straight non-dessert fruit, especially if I am in the mood to eat lots of sweet tasting food.

6.3. Magic of Pectin

Fruits contain pectin, which is magic in the realm of calorie engineering. For instance, consider a box of cake mix. To prepare, I need to add oil and a few eggs. Three ingredients do not give much room to lower down the calories. The oil dwarfs the eggs for calories added. Thanks to the magic of pectin, I can replace oil with applesauce, which is loaded with pectin. This lets me turn a few hundred calories into less than fifty. Each cupcake comes out as fine as a box cake mix can be. I do not notice any difference in the substitution.

Applesauce is the key to my chocolate substitution trick. Many recipes call for chocolate chips or ounces of chocolate. But I like dark chocolate cocoa. I have many recipes where I can use it directly, but sometimes I need to substitute it for chocolate in another recipe. Cocoa mixed with oil and sweetener can substitute for chocolate. I use zero calorie sweetener, but the oil is a major source of calories. Enough to make it more calories than regular chocolate chips. Here is where applesauce comes to the rescue. It replaces the oil. I then get a lower calorie dark chocolate dessert.

Applesauce can replace the oil or butter in any baking recipe. I like applesauce because it is cheap, easy to use, and very low in calories. I keep bottles of applesauce in my cabinet like I used to keep bottles of oil. However, you can use other fruit sauces, jellies, and jams. They may start to add calories, especially sugar-laden jellies, but oil and butter are not hard to beat. I encourage you to experiment and see what you like. I imagine that vanilla cake made with low-sugar strawberry jam would taste good and beat the original calories.

Ice cream was a major component of my obesity. Fruit was there to rescue me from ice cream too. Frozen bananas run through a food processor have the same taste and consistency as ice cream. As you run them, they become crumbly, oatmeal like, and finally ice cream. Optionally you can add in milk, yogurt, or sweetener to get even closer to ice cream. I buy extra bananas each week to freeze. Once I build up a batch, I run them through the food processor. Frozen, blended bananas are what I call ice cream today.

The different stages of texture of grinding the fruit are worth exploring. Each has its own taste. Moreover, you can do the same with other fruits. My wife likes cherries blended in. Meanwhile, frozen strawberries at the crumbly stage feels like I am eating some futuristic form of ice cream.

For the longest time, I tried to get by in life with a food processor or a blender, but not both. Thus, I will make a note of the two in this ice cream regard. It does need to be a food processor to turn frozen banana into ice cream. A blender requires too much liquid to chop it up. But a blender excels at turning frozen fruit into shakes and smoothies, which add lots of liquid. I have and use both devices. They are close, but do not substitute for each other. I recommend getting both as you explore calorie engineering.

6.4. Load up Veggies

When I made spaghetti, it was meat and tomato sauce. It was better on calories than other foods, like pizza. But I asked if I could make it better on calories. At first, I added related vegetables, like onions and celery. Those enhanced the flavor and lowered the calorie density. Then summer hit and I had fresh vegetables flowing into the house, so I added them. I added bell peppers first, and then carrots and squash the next time. My spaghetti has the nutritional profile of a vegetable stew. Yet the aroma and taste make me feel like I am eating by the sea side in Italy. This is the core of how I cook. Take a food, add vegetables, lower the calorie density, and increase the taste and healthiness.

Sloppy Joes are in my standard monthly calendar rotation for dinner. They have much in common with spaghetti sauce, based on meat and tomato sauce. The calorie risk comes from the add-ins of bread and cheese. Spaghetti sauce expects a vegetable melody. There are more recipes I make available online. Sloppy Joes are more traditional with less variety in the added vegetables. Still, I added other vegetables, like carrots, squash, and rice. It was Sloppy Joes version 2.0, with the vegetables making it better. I encourage you to take whatever you make and add more vegetables into it. Even if they do not seem to fit at first, start with a small amount and experiment.

Then there are things like hamburgers. The meat patty can only handle a few added vegetables. Too many turns it into meatloaf, which is not bad in itself, but it is a different food. Remember hamburgers are a delicacy in their own right. I load up my hamburger with vegetables on top of it. I use onions, jalapeños, bell peppers, tomatoes, and as much lettuce as I smash down into the sandwich. My concept is salad crossed with a cheeseburger. It becomes more filling and less calorie dense. The hamburger looks and feels like it will cost you thousands of calories when you pick it up. Same thing works for pizza with vegetable toppings. Anything that cannot be mixed directly with vegetables can be topped with vegetables.

I used to make tacos with Mexican rice as a side. Both were good. However, after every meal, I would have a bowl of left over rice, but no left over taco filling. I combined the two by taking all of the ingredients of both and blending together. These taste so good I have to force myself not to keep having them every week. I save on dish washing too. I do not have to use a separate pot for the rice. Parboiled brown rice cooks up in the same pan with the taco filling and other ingredients. Instead of making vegetables as a side you will not eat, mix them into the main entrée you are eating.

Then there are meals like steak. I cannot mix vegetables into the steak and cannot top it like a hamburger. Vegetables are the side item in those meals. But, who wants to eat vegetables? Thus, I asked "How can I be comfortable eating vegetables as a side?" First, I thought of deep fried French fries. They are a vegetable, but the deep frying triples the potato calories. Next, I thought of my second vegetable love - sweet corn. I grow sweet corn. There is no cost analysis that justifies the effort to grow it for the yield. But I keep growing it for the taste of garden fresh corn. Of course, I was using more butter than corn. Why take the effort to grow sweet if I will bathe it in butter? I can do that with canned corn. In fact, one holiday in winter, I was out of home grown corn and used canned corn. My mother-in-law called it the best corn she ever ate because of how much butter was in it. Overtime, I lowered the butter until it was under control. Now I think of it as mayo, BBQ sauce, and the other add-ins that detract from the main food. Butter is an accent, rather than the main course.

I looked for ways to eat more vegetables. Sweet corn served as my base. I added in a small amount of carrots and peas. I cooked it the same way - steaming hot with butter and salt. It added variety to my meal. Now corn by itself without other vegetables comes off as dull. The best day in my history of eating corn was when I mixed in jalapeños.

A whole tomato is about the same calories as a tablespoon of ketchup. Neither is high calorie. But one tomato takes up so much room on a sandwich that it falls off. I am getting a treat with all the tomato that I can load up on a sandwich. When they are in season during the summer I substitute tomato for ketchup. It is not a big savings. But I save a bit, add variety, and get to eat a sandwich that requires two hands to hold.

When I make a hamburger after work, I want to eat it as soon as it is cooked. I do not feel in the mood to peel and slice up a whole onion sitting on the counter just to add a few pieces. But if I have the onion already cut in pieces in the freezer, then I will add onion. I wash and cut up my vegetables the same weekend I buy them from the grocery store. They wait in the freezer or fridge on standby for when I need them.

For dry beans, I buy a pound, soak overnight, and boil the next morning. Then I freeze portions in freezer bags. You could buy canned beans to save on time. It is only slightly more expensive, but then you have lowered the taste and have to check if they added sugar.

Brown rice takes as long as dry beans to cook. Fortunately, it comes in two versions, and I keep both on hand. First, I use regular brown rice in anything I will be cooking for a long time, such as in the slow cooker. Meanwhile, parboiled brown rice cooks within ten minutes. Whenever I am cooking tacos in a skillet or anything else quick-cooking, I add parboiled brown rice. You could save the extra fifty cents parboiled rice costs. Do the same trick with the dry beans - boil a big pot and freeze portions. More to the point, think about the vegetables that you eat and how to keep those ready to use. If you do not eat beans or rice yet, then do not worry about having them ready to use.

Vegetables are as cheap as the dirt they are grown in. They come frozen, canned, dried, and fresh. The taste varies by vegetable and use. When in season, sweet corn from a local farm will be best to buy if you are not growing it yourself. Second to that is frozen in the grocery store.

The fresh sweet corn in most grocery stores is a few days old and frozen will taste better. Vegetables come in different states of readiness. On this one, most of the time I buy the least processed version and do the prep work myself. But sometimes I buy carrots that are already peeled if I will use them that day and do not feel in the mood to peel a bunch. The nice thing about the extra cost in splurging is they still cost less than processed food.

6.5. Beverages

Drinking and eating are inseparable. Maybe I go a few bites before a drink, but I drink during the entire meal. Even if I have a pop flavor I hate without another drink choice, I end up drinking multiple glasses. That is what makes drinks with high calories dangerous. I used to have a whole meal's worth of calories during the day just from what I drank.

The healthy drinks can deceive. For many years, I drank juice instead of pop. I bought gallons of juice each week instead of cases of pop. I thought I was doing myself a favor, but I was fat the whole time. The reason is simple. Sugar comes from plants, typically vegetables, like beets or corn. Juice comes from plants too, typically fruits, which are higher in sugar than vegetables. Juice is the liquid version of a bag of sugar. As with any sugar, I try to control the amount.

I had friends who were masters of social drinking, but I have been witness to family who ruin their lives with liquor. The latter has left me reluctant to drink liquor often. I could share my own stories, but now I only do it every blue moon every blue year. The last time I was tempted to drink was a New Year's Eve. My wife and I planned to share a bottle of wine. But, I looked up the calories and discovered there were over a hundred calories in a single glass of wine. I then opted to go for a bowl of ice cream instead. If I spend the calories, I want to feel like I am getting something out of it. I feel lucky because if I had been a drinker, then I would have been up at least two more pants sizes.

If you cannot drink pop, juice, or beer with your food, then what do you drink? First, I focused on drinking more water. I know some people who do not drink water. They have become so addicted to chemical drinks they refuse to drink plain water. I was never that bad, so for me, it was more water. If you have to start with drinking water as a new concept, then phase it in over time.

While I might not have been in the no water camp, I was halfway there and needed something to replace that other half. I shifted into diet pop with my meals. Diet pop comes in the same flavors and more. I noticed a slight taste difference. But after a few cans and hundreds of calories saved, the taste grew on me. I set out to try different flavors to add variety. I discovered I liked the fruit flavors the best and after a few months could not stand the plan cola taste. Around Thanksgiving, I tried diet cranberry pop. I do not like cranberry sauce, but diet cranberry pop became my favorite diet pop flavor.

Then I discovered tea. It offered a mix of flavors in a new frontier. I prefer black tea and flavored teas. My cabinet has ten different flavors of tea right now. I always try new ones. I feel like I can go my whole life trying new teas.

Over a few months, tea replaced pop for me. It is cheaper which appeals to my native cheapskate tendencies. Pop tastes terrible to me now. It comes across as an artificial chemical taste, but tea comes across as natural tasting. This reflects the processed nature of the ingredients. Pop is water with the last advancements in chemistry. Meanwhile, tea is leaves and bark scraped off a plant. Processing consists of drying, maybe removing caffeine, and packaging. It appeals to my native love for non-processed foods. Last, I suspect a flavonoid was invented by the tea industry and do not know if tea has health benefits or not. In contrast, there is zero chance that zero calorie soft drinks help my health. I will not be surprised if diet pop comes out as bad for my health. As for the time to prepare tea, it requires boiling water. Or, I can make cold brewed tea overnight in the fridge if I do not feel like taking the time to boil water. There is not a metric I can find that pop has going for it over tea. Yet, I hated tea at first and would never have imagined myself drinking it every day. It was one of the foods I developed a preference for as my tastes sharpened.

The one caution on tea is added sweetener. I use a tablespoon of calorie free sucralose for each half gallon of tea. This makes for a calorie free drink I can enjoy with any meal. Though, I have been meaning to explore adding honey. As long as the sugar level is low, I am not concerned on the calories. I do not think every drink with my meal has to be zero calories, only low calorie. I can spare ten calories in drinks with my meal, but I cannot spare a hundred. Not with my meal at least.

Tonight, after dinner, I ran frozen strawberry, frozen banana, greek yogurt, cocoa, almond milk, and sweetener through a blender. It had no ice cream, but the yogurt brought diary that made it like a milk shake. The dark chocolate cocoa made it better than any chocolate candy, and the strawberry flavor added an accent. My toddler climbs into his high chair to have some. It is one of my favorite drinks and comes in at a fraction of the calories of any ice cream milk shake. I have more shakes and smoothies than ever before. As I said, I avoid high calorie drinks with meals, but I see no reason they cannot be my dessert. A shake is like apple crisp or any other dessert. It is not something to be avoided, but rather something to plan into my daily calorie plan. The enjoyment of my shake would have been lost if I was eating it with dinner, but spacing it out after dinner as its own item ensured full enjoyment. If you do want to drink items with calories, then that is how I suggest you do it. Moreover, everything I said about optimizing the calories apply. For instance, fruit is the center in my shakes and smoothies.

6.6. Cart of Dairy

On my grocery trip today I bought whole milk, two percent milk, unsweetened almond milk, block cheese, sliced cheese, cream butter, margarine, regular cream cheese, and fat-free cream cheese. My cart was a sampler pack of the dairy the store has to offer. Even that description understated it. I made yogurt from the milk, and I had left over sour cream and cultured buttermilk at home from last week. I go through enough dairy that I am tempted to get a cow one day.

The whole milk is for my children, and I will quit buying it once they get older. But for now, we go through at least a gallon of whole milk in one week. It is only twenty calories per cup more than two percent milk. On one hand, that is not much to worry about. But, when I use whole milk in place of two percent milk, I do not see a difference. I can get the vitamin D advertised in whole milk either in almond milk, a multivitamin, or from spending time outside in the sun. I do not feel like I am getting anything for spending those extra twenty calories. If money was tight or we were wasting it, then I would shift to this type of milk.

Before our second child, there would be one week every month where we had a few cups of whole milk left as it hit the expiration date. I started to look for ways to use it. Making yogurt for the children is an easy one. I have even used it my own yogurt. Mixing a small amount into a bigger batch does not impact calories by much. I have also substituted for two percent milk by equal calories. For instance, 1 3/4 cup of two percent milk is about the same calories as 1 1/2 cups of whole milk. Yet, sometimes I have plenty of yogurt and nothing that needs milk. When that happens, I dump it out. I am happy to try to find legitimate ways to use things before they go bad, but I do not consume it just because it is going bad.

The first few months I ate store-bought cereal for breakfast with two percent milk added. I used my prior advice to start looking at the other items near milk in the grocery store. I saw almond milk. I thought of it as a joke. How can an almond have milk? But as I tried out other foods over months, I decided to give it a try. I was surprised when I added it into my store-bought cereal. I did not notice much of a difference. Store-bought cereal carries so much sugar that it sweetens up anything. I could have substituted water and not noticed. Still, this was helpful. It provided a gateway to start using almond milk more and a way to develop a taste for it. Almond milk is now a regular in my household.

Almond milk comes in shades of sugar added: sweetened, light, and unsweetened. At the fully sweetened end, it is near the same calories as cow milk, and I see no point. I purchase the unsweetened variety. I use it as an ingredient in other things, such as mashed potatoes. I do not need any sweetener for those sorts of uses. When I do use it in something like a bowl of homemade granola, I sweeten it myself. This lets me control how much and what kind of sweetener I use. Then I have the flexibility to mix and match sugar and calorie-free sweeteners.

I kept experimenting and trying to substitute almond milk for cow's milk. It has worked out for the majority of substitutions, such as with granola and in fruit shakes. But, I have noticed a few cautions. I made an egg omelet using almond milk. Eggs have a light flavor, and the almond taste dominated. It was not bad, just different. Probably because egg omelets go back to my childhood when my mom made them for me. I am sensitive to change in dear foods. I could have done more to explore working it in, but I did not bother, since my omelet uses only two tablespoons of milk. A ten calorie difference is not worth my time. Meanwhile, the majority of the time there is no taste difference. Other times, it may change the color. I use almond milk in my mashed potatoes. The color is an off-white instead of a creamy white, but no taste difference.

 I eat yogurt like I used to eat ice cream. It is a main stay of every breakfast I have. I tried both whole and two percent milk and did not notice a difference. But, I did not like skim milk based. Thus, I use two percent milk. I use two percent milk for the protein. I could explore almond milk yogurt. With the calories savings, I would be able to eat it in the quantities I used to eat ice cream, but I would lose a good breakfast protein source. I could even do more to give skim milk more of a chance. That would let me save a few calories and keep the protein. But, two percent based fits like a puzzle piece into my daily calorie plan. I see food as providing nutriment. Once it fits into my calories, I do not need to engineer it anymore. I want to knock out the calories that offer nothing, but leave the ones that do.

 A cup of cream, a half pound of butter, and a cup of sugar read like classic cookbook dessert porn. High calorie items team up together. I take aim at each one in turn. I replace the butter with margarine and switch out half the sugar with a calorie-free sweetener. But what about the cream? Most recipes that call for cream do not need it. I do not want to start buying a fourth kind of milk each week. (Technically fifth if you count the powered buttermilk I use in baking.) I do not notice the cream through the butter and sugar. When I go to make something like regular ice cream that calls for cream, I explore options. I may use regular milk, yogurt, or even almond milk. Any recipe that calls for any sort of dairy is open to interruption. Do not restrict yourself to exactly what is being requested. Engineers experiment. Not all things will be great, but chances are they will be good. And being afraid of making a mistake will block you from discovering successes.

I make sourdough bagels with cinnamon added to the dough. Throughout my life, I have never eaten a bagel alone. I eat it with cream cheese. Not doing so is like eating popcorn without butter and salt. Yet, the bagel is heavy on calories from the flour, and the cream cheese can be even more calories. What to do? I have used fat-free cream cheese. The fat-free cream cheese comes in at ketchup level calories and functions like ketchup for bagels. Yet, fat-free cream cheese is lacking for everything else I use cream cheese in, such as cheesecakes. I use either regular cream cheese or reduced fat cream cheese for cheesecake. But where I want a minor accent, the fat-free cream cheese fits.

I used to wash down a big breakfast with glasses of whole milk. I thought I was being healthy. I am lucky no one told me cream was healthier or my pants would have been bigger. As with other high calorie beverages, I quit drinking it with my meals. But I have not quit drinking milk. I still drink multiple glasses of milk. I make shakes, hot cocoa, and smoothies a few times a week. I use almond milk and yogurt in the shakes, and two percent milk in the hot cocoa. I mix and match the dairy to suite. It is a combination of finding what I like and meeting the calories I aiming for. Once I hit that, I am done, and it is onto other calorie challenges.

6.7. Sugar

I joke that I should get a cow with how much dairy my family uses, but I have a beehive in the backyard supplying us with honey. Sugar, what would we do without it? I was deciding which pancake syrup to buy. There was one bottle that proclaimed in loud letters "No High Fructose Corn Syrup." I turned to the ingredient list. The first ingredient was corn syrup. When I see labels like that, I regret shopping at grocery stores. Evaporated cane juice, brown sugar, molasses, honey, rice fructose, corn syrup, and a million others are sugar. These are extracted from nature and dropped in a package. Then they hire a drunken writer to make up words for the label: fat-free, healthy, organic, or natural. Sugar is to the food industry like a packaging box is to my toddler: endless loads of fun.

The sugar added to food is important to me. However, I could not tell you how many grams of sugar are in the foods I eat. I do not look at the grams of sugar. I look at the total calories, which will be high if it is high in sugar, and I look at the ingredient list. I look for sugar early in the list and multiple forms of sugar.

Is there a health difference between corn syrup, honey, or beet sugar? When I was north of three hundred pounds, I wasted many hours researching that question. It was like trying to research how to be the world's champ at Tic-Tac-Toe. The real question: Is there a health difference between being obese and the type of sugar I eat? Obesity has been proving bad for both quality and length of life. Meanwhile, debates about forms of sugar fill online discussions. Now that obesity is behind me, I tell myself the honey from my own beehive is healthier than every other form of sugar. Who knows if it is true. But I am no longer choosing between types of sugar and obesity. And when I go to use that honey, I am honest with myself on the calories in it - sixty four calories per tablespoon. That number hits my mind before I lift the lid off the jar.

Sugar in small quantities, like salt, enhances the food and is needed for many desserts. What to do? When I first started, I declared war on sugar. It was a war that I won and lost battles on. I do not regret waging the war because it was key to getting me to where I am. But sugar ranks a mere pawn in the obesity war.

My first strategy was to make greater use of calorie-free sweeteners. I have no particular preference for the different calorie-free forms. I purchase bulk generic sucralose because it is cheapest. I may take a try at growing Stevia, since I garden, but my use would eclipse however much I could grow. In most desserts, I started using half regular sugar and half calorie-free. Then I tried shifting the balance more towards calorie-free sweeteners. In any drinks, like tea, I only use calorie-free sweetener. Even brown sugar can be substituted. I use one tablespoon of molasses to one cup of calorie-free sweetener.

It was not costing me calories, but it felt I was still hooked on a different form of sugar. Calorie-free sweeteners are part of the answer, but they are not the entire answer. They are expensive and processed wonders of chemical wizardry. Today, I blend regular forms of sugar with a calorie-free sweetener, but I quit trying to shift the balance beyond half and half. Except in drinks I have with meals, like tea. My new approach is to lower the total amount of sweetener, calorie-free or not. This is easier now that my tastes are sharper. It might not be something you can do in the first few months, but looking back, I could have started this approach sooner. I take whatever I am making and try to work the sweetener down to a reasonable level. Each time I make it, I use a little less until I feel the calories fit or the sweetener level feels right. For instance, my favorite chocolate cake recipe uses two tablespoons each of honey and sucralose and comes out to two hundred twenty five calories per serving. I never tried lowering the sweetener further because it fits my calorie budget at that level.

Chocolate cake and any other foods need sweetener added, and not just a dash. My cake recipe needs two tablespoons of sugar and below that it is not worth eating. The minimum amount needed is personal and changes. I needed closer to two cups instead of two tablespoons in my cake recipe when I started this journey. The level needed in cake and other foods dropped with the pounds. Once I hit the minimum amount of sweetener, I can keep adding more sugar. It may taste better, but the calorie and taste return start to drop. I could double the honey in my chocolate cake recipe. I would add over a hundred calories, but it would not taste a hundred calories better. To get my chocolate cake up to winning a food contest at an obesity convention would require over two cups of sugar. But again, the return on the calories is not there for me at the obesity reformist convention. I look for balance where food tastes good and leads my tastes to lower sweetener levels. My new fruit habit helped too. I did not realize it as such, but using fruit is a way to cut down on added sweeteners. Fruit comes with sugar packaged inside, plus fiber and nutrients. It is an actual food.

6.8. Bread

Bread and I have a modern-day relationship. We have spent time together, separated, and seen others. When I was fat, I ate every form of bread I could find. I bought store-bought junk bread, often falling for anything labeled healthy or ancient. I made homemade bread loaded with sugar and butter. Whenever I visited Chicago, I made sure to stop by an authentic deep dish pizza parlor to get a hit of the pizza crust. Bread ranked with ice cream and mayo in my top five sources of overeating calories.

As I mentioned, the size of the buns I used were out of control in portion size. I switched to sliced bread for hamburgers and sandwiches, but it was still a calorie sink. I upgraded to thirty-five calorie per slice bread. When I did, two hamburgers for dinner was not a calorie breaker. I stayed with light sliced bread for most of my weight loss journey. From time to time, I tried regular sliced bread and even regular buns. They did not taste better. I am willing to spend more calories, but I want a return on them to make it worthwhile.

Sloppy Joes earn their name when I try to eat them on a bun. Even the largest bun made of the most ancient grains cannot hold up. But the bread is an accent, not a main player. The big pot of tomatoes, peppers, and seasoning is the main player. Trying to make the bread the main player equals eating tomato flavored wads of bread. Thus, I eat it with a fork as an open-face sandwich. I plow the calories saved into more filling and better bread. Plus, I have enough to sprinkle sharp cheddar cheese on top which I can taste without the bread getting in the way.

For pizza, sliced bread does not substitute for pizza crust. There is the standard pizza crust and thin varieties, but I learned I have even other choices beyond those. First, at the low calorie end, I replaced the crust with flat bread tortilla shells. Those let me eat pizza within my calories goals before I knew how to get any other component of the pizza under control. I was eating flat bread pizzas every week when I started. Switching out the pizza bread was easier to start with than taking on the cheese and other aspects of the pizza, which I was able to do later on. At the other end, I have taken baguettes and torn out the filling in the center, then made French bread pizza. The tearing-out the center filling of baguettes and buns is a useful method for anytime you use bread.

Baking has been one of my hobbies of which I have felt most proud because it is hard and not as many dare to try it. But, I took a break from baking as I set out on this journey. I debated about starting to bake again. I wondered if doing so would put me back to obese. But I realized where I had gone wrong. I baked as if I was making candy. I made homemade rolls, bagels, and other items but bought the same sorts of breads at the grocery store. Baking was not a calorie replacement, but a calorie addition source. Once I realized that, I changed it to fit my engineering needs. Today, I bake to replace what I would have bought at the grocery store. I quit buying buns, loaf bread, bagels, and other breads that I make at home. Every weekend, I make a batch of homemade buns to use for the next week.

As I went back into baking, I wanted something more than the sugar and butter infused breads I used to eat. I sat out to learn to make sourdough bread. Full mastery will take decades of experience. But long before then, sourdough brings a world of flavors, tastes, and novelty. The bread derives flavor notes from the sourdough aspect without requiring heaps of other add-ins. I use my homemade buns for my hamburgers, peanut butter sandwiches, and everything else. They are higher calories than light sliced bread. But they bring new flavor notes and are like adding another variety item to the meal. Now that I have got the other components under calorie control I can afford to spend more for a bun worthy of its weight in calories. My light bread phase was still useful. At the time, bread controlled me and light bread helped get me to where I controlled bread.

Moreover, I bake with white whole wheat flour. It is whole wheat, the white prefix only means a lighter form of wheat was used. I do not find the need to use cake flour, bread flour, or others. I find white whole wheat close enough for the job. Sourdough lends natural to whole wheat breads because baker's yeast cannot handle rising it.

Chapter 7: Dining In and Out

"If you set out to be liked, you would be prepared to compromise on anything at any time, and you would achieve nothing." - Margaret Thatcher

7.1. Where to Eat Out

I can eat pizza, steak, hamburgers, fried chicken, taco, and ice cream with sprinkles in one place, as much as I want, for one price. The call of a buffet is like the sirens call in the sea. I have been lured to my doom there more times than I care to admit. Even reading my sentence, it sounds appealing, but I know it tastes mediocre. On days I went to the buffet, I would try to avoid eating before going, trying to maximize my buffet value. When I went, I stuffed myself until I could barely waddle out the door. Yet, later in the day, I would be hungry again. Then I would get the sick buffet hangover for at least the rest of the day if not the next. The buffet is a dream that never materializes. Worse, I thought the more I ate at the buffet, the better the deal I was getting. The deal I got was worse health. I would have been better off paying the buffet to not give me any food. I would have earned my money back in medical bills.

Now when I dine out, I favor restaurants that are better on calories. Mexican restaurants work the best for me and I enjoy the spicy foods. The time I spent in New Mexico was the best restaurant eating period of my life. A full meal and sides is not much more than my home cooked dinner.

I did not give up the high calorie restaurants. I rotate in lower calories ones more often. Except for buffets, I aim to never eat a plate again that has tacos with a side of pizza and a side of ice cream on the other side. This left me in need of a substitute for buffet restaurants. Two towns over, I found it. It was a cafeteria style restaurant with people lined out the door into the parking lot. They have a wide selection of the popular foods, but they sell by the item instead of an entry fee. This provides benefits for both the restaurant and me. First, I never felt like I had to eat extra food for my money's worth. Moreover, since a slice of cheesecake and a roll are different prices, they can make each item better. At the buffet, it is scary because the fried chicken and hamburgers taste the same. At the cafeteria restaurant, fried chicken tastes like fried chicken, not everything else they are selling. Last, I have never had the buffet hangover. I would dine there more often if it were not for the waiting line. Others are in on the secret.

When I was not going to a buffet, I picked a restaurant that served unlimited rolls. I ate rolls before the food got there, with the food, and after I was done eating my meal. There was two meals worth of calories in rolls alone. As a change, I minimized temptation by picking restaurants without unlimited rolls. When I ventured back to those places, I was on guard. I am willing to spend calories on bread if it is good. But even then I am careful because it is high calorie and comes with a delayed full feeling. I used to eat four rolls before the main entrée arrived. Now I let the rolls sit until I am served the main course. Then, I eat the roll with the food or after. The last such restaurant I went to, I ate a single roll over the course of the whole dinner. Considering how many rolls I used to eat that feat is one of the top achievements of my life.

Salsa and tortilla chips are on an unlimited free tap at Mexican restaurants. I like those, but not as much as rolls. Even when I was obese, I did not have the same addiction to them as I did with rolls. If I had cheese dip with the tortillas, then I would overeat it. But cheese dip is an appetizer you have to buy separate, so no buffet syndrome risk.

7.2. What to Order Out

A local Italian restaurant was advertising a new low calorie pasta entrée. It was on the TV commercials and plastered all over the building doors. It was not my reason for going, but I could not help but miss their new offering. As I looked around, I spotted a sign in the back for the staff. "Try to upgrade the light pasta to the large with extra cheese." I wondered how many people had been victimized by that scheme. I was not that day, but I had been in the past. The light entrées are often there to bait people in. Then they try to push a bigger size and more add-ons, like extra cheese. You are left with an entrée that resembles nothing of the low calorie version.

I have made plenty of mistakes at restaurants. I saw chicken pot pie on the menu. I thought it would have the calorie profile of chicken, vegetables, and other items added. After the meal, I researched. I discovered I was off by a thousand calories. It was crust, butter, oil, and other items added. Chicken and vegetables fell into the other items part. On a different occasion, I thought I was being healthy and calorie conscience when I ordered green beans as a side with my steak. The green beans had enough butter dumped into them that my toddler would have eaten them. Restaurants do not make the food in a low or even medium calorie way. They make it in the highest possible calorie way that appeals to the widest part of the population which helps them stay the widest.

Even at safer restaurants, I pay attention to the menu and do my calorie math. On a recent visit, the chicken enchiladas were a hundred calories less than the beef enchiladas. I do not notice a difference between beef and chicken when it is wrapped with a tortilla and covered with cheese and sauce. Beneath those two choices was a third labeled "skinny chicken enchiladas." It was over two hundred calories less than the regular chicken. The description said they used water instead of oil to soften the tortillas and ranchero sauce instead of cream cheese sauce. My side item choices were refried beans, black beans or rice. Refried beans are my common choice. However, they were a hundred calories more than the rice and fifty calories more than the black beans. I would have made that switch, but I did not need to. The refried beans and skinny chicken enchiladas together fit into the calories I wanted to spend for dinner.

Appetizers and desserts are obesity bait. I cannot think of a time when I needed the extra calories to round out my meal. My wife sometimes orders an appetizer as the dinner entrée since they come in such big portions.

When I was obese, I never took home leftovers, except for a stash of extra rolls I would ask for before going. If seven chicken strips were served, then I ate seven chicken strips, even if I was content at five. Today, when the calories will be over what I want to spend, I ask for a to-go box up front. Planning to use a to-go box frees me up from eating whatever I am served. I eat until I am good, then take the rest to-go. This is also an inner toddler trick, do not eat food just because it is placed in front of you.

7.3. Eating like Lemmings

Lemmings are cute little creatures with a reputation for jumping off cliffs in big packs. Back when I was younger, I spent many hours playing a video game based on lemmings. The goal was to keep the lemmings out of trouble - no matter how much they tried to jump off the cliff together. In the game, each lemming would follow the next, repeating the same mistake and running into the same danger. When I eat with a group, I feel like one of those eight bit lemmings back in my video game. The larger the group, the more special the occasion, the worse it is. The appetizers, desserts, entrées, and drinks appear like bonus items in a video game. Even if I want none, I feel like the right thing to do is to follow the crowd. I needed to break out of the lemmings pack, but not reveal myself to be a non-lemming.

Talking comes a close second to jumping off the eating cliff together. Any group gathering should be more about the people than about the food, but often we let the food dominate. Try to talk to, listen to, and experience others as much as experiencing the food. Discussing the weather, what brought everyone together, and what everyone has been up to are conversation appetizers. If I keep in mind that I am trying to talk more than eat, then it helps me. However, if I do not pay attention, then the food can flow as easily as the words.

Once, after eating with a large group, the next day some of them said, "Sorry for making you go over your calories last night". I told them, "Not to worry. It is an average." That is true for a one-off day, but I was more strategic than that. During the meal, I chopped up my food and shifted it around on the plate. I dumped ketchup and waded up napkins on the plate. I ate half my food, but the plate looked like it was ready for the track. No one else noticed. If they did, then they would have thought I was channeling my inner toddler. They would have been right.

One of my friends knows one alcoholic drink will never be enough for him. Whenever he is out with people, he tells them he cannot drink because of some medication he is taking. He tells himself that too, even though it is not true. If they ask questions, he will mention a side effect about getting sick. From that point forward, the group helps him not to drink. The same approach can work with food. The world of medical pills is ever expanding with long precautions about what not to eat or take with them. For instance, if you are on blood thinners, you need to avoid dark leafy green vegetables. That can be a reason for avoiding the salad dressing laden course. Related, there are countless allergies to nuts, diary, and other foods. Any food can be suspect of containing an allergen. Pick one and use that as your excuse for not eating. I hate to advise lying, but I would hate for you to get heart disease more. If you are with a group that understands and you can be honest with them then go ahead and be honest. But I know from experience, there will times when the group is not supportive. At times, you will have fellow fat people who laugh at your attempts to lose weight, or your distant aunt who insists you are nothing but skin and bones.

Going over on calories during a night out, at a birthday party, or for a big holiday will not hurt your overall efforts. A single day becomes a wash amongst the other days. The average is what drives your weight. When it becomes once a week or more often, that is where the danger is.

The ideal situation would be to dine-out without temptation of going over on calories. Try to fit it into your calorie plan. Then you can go out every day if you want. I can do that at the right places with one or two others. But when marching with the lemmings to an unknown cliff, I am at risk of falling.

When all else fails, I avoid the lemming march, especially for lunch gatherings. The middle of the day is a terrible time for me to overeat. No matter how big lunch is, I will be hungry later in the day. I am relaxed on dinner because I will be in bed a few hours after. Of course, there is a danger in avoiding too many group gatherings, and I have made that mistake sometimes. But in finding stability in a new lifestyle, skipping a few food gatherings is not that bad.

Not everything is a preplanned gathering. Wherever there are people, there is food. A friend at work brought in bagels. She offered me "carb-free" bagels then laughed. Two years ago if someone passed me a bagel, they would have the cream cheese in the other hand. At the start, it was hard to say no to the first bagel. But after twenty times, I do not have to lift my fingers from the keyboard to say no. With each no, the habit grows and others understand your new habit.

Of course, if bagels are regular at work on Friday, then you can build that into your calorie plan for Friday and enjoy one. The key is to set the limit to an amount that fits into your calories and plan for it. Make sure the bagel you allow yourself is not your first step down the lemming cliff.

7.4. How It Is Cooked

I cooked chicken like I was harboring a traumatic childhood experience with raw chicken. The chicken came out so dry it needed gobs of mayo to rescue it. That worked for me when I was obese, but I needed to reduce mayo to a background accent. That cannot happen if the chicken is dry as rock. I started making it using a meat thermometer to be precise as to when it was done. Since I had been guessing, I had to leave a safety net. Thermometer use requires keeping a close watch. My house is full of pint-sized distractions getting into everything. Chicken takes a half-hour to reach halfway done, and a few minutes to turn to rock after that. As a solution, I marinated the chicken overnight. It provided a buffer against overcooking and added flavor notes. Marinades turned out to fit well into my week. I make homemade Greek yogurt twice a week. The leftover whey makes a good marinade. Most of the time I dump it out, but if I have something to marinade I use it.

I constructed lasagna as layers of cheese with filling in between. Yet the cheese flavor was lost amiss the sauce and other ingredients. This led me to try ever greater amounts of cheese. When I broke the recipe into calorie sources, I saw I was eating a tray of cheese that tasted like spaghetti sauce. Then I removed the cheese from the middle layers and put it on top. The lasagna had the visual of a cheese lover's delight. The fork carried a burst of cheese flavored lasagna. Moreover, I did not need as much cheese because even a small amount shined bright. I saved hundreds of calories.

When I cooked my first black bean veggie burger, I pan fried it in at least a quarter cup of olive oil. The taste made me think vegetation eating could be tasty. I congratulated myself on using healthy olive oil. Then when I paid attention to calories, I learned the oil made it higher in calories than any beef burger I made. Whenever I pan fried, I was eating more calories from the oil than the intended food. Thus early on, I got scared off pan frying, and I avoided it until I felt more in control. Then I started again using small amounts of oil. I start with a tablespoon and adjust from there. The black bean burger does not taste as ultimate as I remember from my obese days, but still has a good flavor profile. The other foods I was eating like fried eggs still taste good. I am eating buttery fried eggs instead of eggy melted butter. And sometimes I pan fry meat and finish it in the oven. As long as I keep a watch on the oil, it works for me.

The deep fryer was the sea where my meals came from. I would bread meat or chicken and drop them in. Even prepared food was a victim. The manufacturer deep fries pizza rolls before packing, but I deep fried them to heat them up. To my obese self, it tasted like perfection. A turkey deep fryer seemed the key to more pleasure, but I held back. The oil costs more than a turkey. My inner cheapskate saved me a pant size.

A deep fryer is harder to clean than a neglected microwave. Even when I was obese that made me think twice in using it. Now with sharper tastes, the cleaning is not justified. Deep fried food tastes like grease and I feel like I lose hundreds of calories. Even if I get nostalgic, I am stopped at the calorie calculation. No one can tell me how to calculate calories for deep frying, which is fitting. I pan fry in moderation, but I will never have need to clean a deep fryer again.

A world without a deep fryer does not mean a world without French fries. Bring a pot of water to a boil. Add a spoonful of baking soda into it. Cut up potatoes into slices and boil for about four minutes. Enough to get them hot. Drain. Optionally, add spices. You can even add a small amount of oil or butter to the slices. Bake at 450 degrees until done. Cooking in a convection oven or a cooling rack will get it crispier. No oil mess and calories come from the potatoes. Before, my oven was for baking cookies, but now I bake fries, country steak, and so many other foods. And I pay only for the calories in the potatoes, not the oil. Moreover, using fresh vegetables with spices sharpen the taste more than oil ever could.

A smoker opens even more possibilities to replace oil. I make pulled pork in my smoker every month. I wondered what if I smoked a beef roast and made pulled beef? It had a stronger beef flavor than deep frying and tones of hardwood smoke. It was a new way to cook something I had been making that added no additional calories.

7.5. Defining Portion

Circular plates were not meeting my demands. I would fill it and then had to keep getting up to get refills. I upgraded to square plates and gained the surface area of the missing corners. Then I could add more food. After a few months with my new plates, the amount of food I ate had grown to take up the whole plate. I wondered if I should check for any even bigger plate size or if there was a modern computer-designed shape that might solve the plate surface area problem.

When I found out how many calories where on my square and thought about the refills, I decided to move in the opposite direction. I went back to the circular plates. At first, it felt like a kid's sized plate. After a few weeks, I did not think about it.

I still use my original circular plates for dinner, but they feel large for other meals and snacks. I bought a collection of smaller plates for lunch, and even a few kids-sized plates for snacks. Getting up to refill the plate helped slow me down and ask myself how many calories into lunch I was. When I committed to the large plate for lunch, I ate the food on the plate. But the smaller plate gave me a chance to ask the "How much to eat?" question as I went without committing up front. On a high calorie danger night, like pizza, I use the lunch plates for dinner to add in that pause for refills.

The old square plates are still in my cabinet and get frequent use. They make for platters to prepare food on. I can layout four slices of bread side by side. Plus I can stack several ears of corn on them as a serving platter. They have become invaluable as I freeze more fruits and meat. One plate holds at least three bananas sliced up, or four quarter-pound hamburger patties. When I need to cut up small amounts of an onion or another vegetable, the plates are there again as a not-so-mini cutting board. These plates have much utility for everything except for eating.

I ate with tall bowls that could hold half a carton of ice cream. Still, I had to choose between room in the bowl for more ice cream or for extra toppings, like sprinkles or candy. I downsized those - the same as I did my plates. I use a normal sized bowl to eat from. Unless it is a low-calorie soup dish because then there was little danger in eating too much. At the other end, I purchased small mixing ingredient bowls that hold a half cup each. They are useful for mixing ingredients, but I get more use as dessert bowls. Each one holds a single serving of ice cream. At the start of my journey, they let me have my visual of a heaping bowl of ice cream.

Why does every silverware set have so many butter knives? They were only used at my house once or twice a year, and that was by a visitor. I used to use spoons for scooping out everything from butter to mayo. I had neglected the butter knife, but it was what I was missing. It is ideal to get the correct serving size of mayo and as the name implies butter. It replaced the spoon as my default measuring and scooping utensil. These days it is not uncommon for me to have many spoons in the silverware drawer and for every butter knife to be dirty.

I could never cut a cake into the dozen servings it provides. A twelfth of a cake looks like a fourth of a cake. Then as I get down to the end, I am trying to cut the last third into nine pieces to balance out to twelve. Worse, eating a fourth of a cake feels like the start of a good snack. Meanwhile, eating three cupcakes seems like many. From cake to brownies, I now make it in my cupcake pan instead of a big tray. Most items are low enough on calories that I can eat two.

The ramekins were sitting in my cabinet with other unused gifts of years past. Then when I confronted my dessert portion problem, I explored using them. They can hold enough of a dessert for me to walk away satisfied. Eating out of one felt like I was eating a miniature cake. I engineer the ingredients and total amount of calories to come out to two to three hundred calories per ramekin. This does not mean cutting down to nothing per ramekin. Take cheesecake; dividing it into that calorie range while using cream cheese is tough and does not quite fill up the whole ramekin. But if I add in strawberries, then it does not add many calories and fills the ramekin to the brim. Plus, the ramekin can go from oven, to table, to fridge, and to microwave. I save dish washing and calories. They rank with butter knives for the prize for "best under used kitchen serving ware."

7.6. How Much to Eat

How much of a food should I eat? What is the right amount? My old answer was if the food fit on the plate, with consumption measured in gobs and fractions of the package it came in. Now, I had calories budgeted for a meal. But, I did not know how much to eat, or how to shift from eating gobs to eating anything that could be measured.

For breakfast, I ate four eggs fried in gobs of butter. I stepped down to three eggs. Once months had passed and I was comfortable, I decreased to two eggs. During the same time, I stepped the butter down a half tablespoon at a time. Each time I went down, I verified I still I liked it. Today when I make fried eggs, I use two eggs and either a tablespoon of margarine or a half tablespoon of cream butter. The way I make fried eggs has remained unchanged for a year. I have enough calories left over to have sausage, sourdough toast, and yogurt mixed with fruit.

There are recommendations about how much meat to eat on a sandwich. They say something about a deck of cards, the size of your palm, or something else that I cannot rationalize. But stepping down a small amount at a time helped me right-size how much meat I use on my sandwiches. Five ounces of meat used to be my minimum amount on a sandwich. Now four ounces of meat is my maximum per sandwich. If I want more than four ounces of meat, like for dinner, then I make a second sandwich. The exact amount depends on how many calories in the kind of meat I am using and what else I am eating with it.

Many recipes call for sticks of butter with many other calorie-laden foods. I ask myself what if I used one less tablespoon of butter? Would I notice? Many recipes call for a stick of butter, but I have never seen a recipe that called for an odd amount, like six and half tablespoons. Yet, saving even one tablespoon of cream butter is a hundred calories that can be regained. People are sticking to the round measurements rather than finding the ideal balance. The ideal amount could be a tablespoon more or less. Might as well experiment with less.

I made my chicken sandwich by taking hunks of chicken breast and putting them on my bun. It would bulge in the middle, lean over the edge, yet still leave pockets of bun without chicken. I engineered a solution - pile on more thick pieces of chicken breast. As I stepped down in my calories, I took another look at my solution. I started chopping up the chicken breast into small pieces and spreading out across the bun. I did not need as many ounces of chicken breast.

A pre-fab slice of cheese is like a sweater your grandmother buys for you. It never fits right, is bulky in some places, and is short in others. Moreover, I could not help but feel cheated on some calories when cheese was lost over the side of the hamburger to the frying pan. But for dinner I make two hamburgers, so I took a single slice and spread it out across two hamburgers. Did not feel cheated, and the cheese more evenly coated the hamburgers.

I bought the candy that came in potato chip sized bags. A bag was as cheap as a value meal, which meant I could get three bags each week. I found myself unwrapping candy whenever I was home, but I did not find enjoyment. It was like I had a candy unwrapping physiologic disorder. When I wanted to reclaim calories, I looked around my kitchen counters and the bags of candy called out. I needed to free up counter space if nothing else.

I switched to premium chocolate candy. It comes in small lunch-sized bags and has triple the cost. This was one of the few times in my life I spent more money on purpose. But it is meant to be eaten one piece at a time, not handfuls at a time. Factoring in cost per serving, then I can still call myself a cheapskate. Most of the manufacturers of the low-end candy peddle candy with premium labels. Those are bags of gourmet sugar and not worth the extra money. I looked for the brands that do not make the low-end too and for better ingredients, like higher cacao levels. With better tasting candy, I did not feel the overeat urge. I ate a piece in the morning after I got to work or on the drive to work. I started hoping for traffic jams on the way to work because it gave me an excuse to eat my morning piece of candy. At home, the bag was stashed on top of the fridge, and when I left for work, I took one piece with me. My routine and keeping it out of sight helped me avoid eating bags at a time. Chocolate was a food I could start with. If I had tried this with ice cream at first, then I would have gained weight and been out more money. That was at first. I could make a change to less of the premium version for anything today. Though on that note, I feel any version of my cheap homemade food is more premium than anything I can buy. But, that comes later.

I prefer a meal that is a rainbow of flavors. I had six ounces of roast chicken cooked on my grill for Sunday dinner. With that I had half a plate of mashed potatoes and a cup of gravy, not the watery kind, but the creamy kind. I ate it with a slice of homemade sourdough bread. Afterward I had a mix of corn, carrots, and jalapeños with half a tablespoon of cream butter. This meal cost me seven hundred calories.

Variety is not only for a meal based on multiple items. It works for a single entrée meal. For instance, I used to eat sandwiches on store bought bread. For a time, I used light bread and had calories left over to spend. Instead of another side item, I upgraded the bread to homemade sourdough bread. It cost me more in calories, but the distinct sourdough bread tones were like adding another side item. Plus not to mention all the veggies I top the sandwich with that further add variety.

Chapter 8: What to Eat

"The doctor of the future will no longer treat the human frame with drugs, but rather will cure and prevent disease with nutrition." - Thomas Edison

8.1. False Choices

Each cereal box has a healthy check mark, list of vitamins, pictures of cartoon characters, and if you are lucky a prize in the box. Cereal would make the high school year book for healthiest food, but this prediction shares the same fate as other yearbook projections. In many grocery stores, cereal and candy share an aisle, and that is the better indicator. The contents of each box are as processed as the rectangular box it is packaged in. It may start with fields of grains and nuts. Then they pulverize it beyond recognition, add filler, and dump in assorted sugars. Enough sugar to burn through your body so you want a second bowl as you finish the last bite of the first. Next, part of a multivitamin goes in, so they can list vitamins as part of the food. If you are worried you are not getting enough vitamins, then take a multivitamin. Some vitamins come with cartoon characters on the package, like the cereal boxes. Thus, you can get your fix of cartoon characters and actual vitamins.

Olive oil is in the top ten list of healthy foods, and I use it. But long before this program, I discovered olive oil and its health benefits. I swapped olive oil for butter in my sweet corn and did not miss the butter. I fried black bean veggie burgers in a pan of olive oil and did not miss the meat. Moreover, olive oil is a liquid and pours out in tablespoons. It screams use me. I bought warehouse club-sized bottles each month. When I looked at calories, I learned olive oil is more calories than butter. Thus, my first step was to switch back from olive oil to butter, and my second step was to switch to margarine. Now that I do not have the urge to overeat, I started using olive oil again. A grocery store sized-bottle lasts me for months.

I thought salads would make me healthier. The trouble was I viewed lettuce as best enjoyed smothered in the grease from a bacon cheeseburger. I discovered a solution to the problem - buttermilk ranch dressing. It makes even tree bark taste good. That was all I needed to start eating a salad before dinner. I prepared a bowl salad mix and gave it a bath in dressing. I began to crave the dressing and started to have it with bread, pizza rolls, and other foods. Lest to say I did not lose any weight from my salad days. When I started this program, I was not much for salads, so I quit trying to work them into my meals. Now I have one on occasion and use no dressing or a small amount. And the hamburgers I make have a salad on top of them without dressing.

I ate an organic apple in the morning and then followed it up with a bagel and cream cheese from the bagel shop. Who knows what GMO food stuffs, additives, pesticides, or chemicals they put into my second course. Likewise, I felt good about my free-range antibiotic-free chicken, but I did not bother asking where the ingredients in my pizza came from. I gained the dual benefits of being both hypocritical and paying attention to the wrong aspect, but no benefits of weight loss.

For every food web search there is a blog talking about how the food you searched for is bad. Meanwhile, there is a good deal of medical research proving obesity steals your health. And in this way, I came to know the truth. What good is a bushel of organic apples if I am a hundred fifty pounds overweight? I did not want to face that one. Switching from eating lots of junk food to lots of healthy foods is as easy asking to super size a happy meal. Meanwhile, facing down changing my lifestyle with food felt beyond me because I did not know this was as easy as it was. Today, calories rein at the top of my healthy food factors above any other fancy terms, labels, or images on the box. I was there to lose weight not eat my way to Zen.

8.2. Whole Grains

Parboiled rice was on sale. The grocery story had it on the top shelf above fifty other less healthy choices. When I was getting a box of brown rice down, a shorter elder woman asked me to get her a box down too. I reached for another box of brown rice, but she said she wanted the white rice. As I handed it to her, I wondered if I had done her a favor. Refined grains are equivalent to eating pure sugar to your body but not your tastes. If I am going to do that, I might as well take a hit of pure sugar and get my enjoyment out of it. Today, I go to lengths to avoid the refined grains. I pick brown rice, old fashion oatmeal, whole wheat tortillas, and whole wheat pasta. Grain-based foods are filling and whole grains ensure the full feeling lasts longer than a half hour.

The calorie difference between whole wheat and refined grain is minor. It may be the same, more, or less. For instance, in one brand I buy, a serving of brown rice has ten calories more than white rice. But, this comparison is like saying a piece of candy has fewer calories than a serving of brown rice. The piece of candy is closer to what the white rice is once your body digests it. Thus, I pick whole grain, even if it is higher in calories.

When I started to look for whole grain products, I saw phrases like "made with whole grain" and "source of whole grain." When I read the ingredients white flour was first on the list. As long as they add a single gram of whole grain, they can stamp a label like that on the box. Another tactic I have seen is the phrase "wheat flour." It does not mean whole wheat but is meant to be mistaken for it.

The marketing gimmicks do not stop there. Down the shelf is ancient grain. People have been growing all grains for thousands of years. How ancient do you need it? Meanwhile, the mixed grain varieties are mixed with white refined grains. These other labels may not even have whole grain in them. They can be refined versions of other grains and comply with their label. Read the ingredient list to know for sure.

I eat whole grains every day and feel good about it. About six percent of the population is sensitive to gluten. I equate this to other food allergies, like a nut allergy. If you have it, then it is no laughing matter and you need to avoid it. But by the way gluten-free is advertised you would think this condition impacted ninety percent of the population. There are whole aisles with gluten-free products. Then throughout the store, foods I did not think would ever have grains as an ingredient, like marshmallows, will have stamps of gluten-free. Why are marshmallows made from pure sugar advertised as gluten-free? To trick people. I know someone who is sensitive to gluten, and he said this works out well for him. For everyone else, it is like avoiding peanuts when you do not have a peanut allergy. If you suspect you have it, then see a doctor to know for sure. It is a serious medical condition, but is not one impacting as much of the population as the food industry advertises.

8.3. Delicious Fat

What if we could create an oil with a long shelf live, that was cheap to manufacture, and tasted good to the masses? Bonus points if it could be re-used several times over for deep frying. Meet partially hydrogenated oil, a wonder of modern mad food science, and the source of trans fat. I avoid it like an obese man avoids a wilderness hike. The Food and Drug administration (FDA) has ruled trans fat is not "generally recognized as safe." With the consequence being what you would expect from the government. The phase out will take place over years and leaves in loop holes. Thus, trans fat will continue to lurk in food.

The best way to identify trans fat food would be a poison label on the side. But that would be too helpful. I have to dig further. First, I check the nutrient food panel for any trans fat. However, food companies are allowed to round down. Thus, 0.49 grams of trans fat per serving can legally be listed as 0 grams per serving. When was the last time you ate a single serving? Especially in the sorts of high calorie foods that have trans fat? Second, I scan through the ingredients looking for partially hydrogenated oil. I ignore fully hydrogenated oil. It is only the partially that is the trans fat concern.

Checking the food ingredient list for the trans fat bogeyman may seem daunting. Most products are not at risk. But certain ones, like peanut butter and frosting, are at risk. Once you get to know these categories, it helps focus your search. Beyond that, I like reading the labels. I am not searching long for trans fat, white flour, or anything else. If it is not obvious what makes up the food, then I do not buy that food.

Add your height and weight together into one number, nothing more complicated. Tell me what that means about your health? That is how useful the total fat on the nutrition panel is. It mixes the trans fat poison with the other kinds. I laugh when I see a bag of marshmallows labeled fat-free. They are made from pure sugar instead. A calorie from sugar puts on the pounds the same as a calorie from fat. The difference is fat is more filling for longer. Moreover, monounsaturated and polyunsaturated fats are good for you, more is better. Subject to calorie limits of course. Peanut butter is a mainstay of my lunch because it is loaded with unsaturated fat.

Meanwhile, saturated fat is fine in moderation. The main source is meat from beef, pork, lamb, or any other mammal. I still eat hamburgers made from beef. For other foods, like chili or tacos, I have switched to turkey or chicken. They are lower calories that way. I try not to eat red meat more than twice a week and my saturated fat intake is fine when I check.

The medical establishment used the term red meat because of the level of myoglobin in the meat. But who knows or cares what myoglobin is? The term red meat is confusing. Pork chops that look white are not what they are talking about when they say white meat. The pork industry tries to capitalize on the misunderstanding. When discussing health or saturated fat in red meats, they mean meats from mammals. Try not to be like I was eating it every day and you should be fine.

8.4. Embrace Whole Foods

Eating processed foods left me feeling like a processed person, but I was prepared to eat them if needed to succeed. I put my calorie needs first. Light margarine was my rebound relationship. It reduced the calories in fried eggs, bowls of popcorn, and ears of sweet corn. I could not have done it without light margarine. It continues to have a place in my heart despite being diluted with water and filled with fake butter chemical compounds. But I would still make the same choice again. Maybe at 120 years old, they will discover light margarine may cause cancer. I can live with that because otherwise I will not live to half that age. Now that the urge to overeat has left, I worked in cream butter and olive oil. I can replace a tablespoon of margarine with a tablespoon of cream butter and not feel cheated. Once when I was obese someone suggested that to me as a technique and I had to laugh. There was no way I could have done that when I was obese. I still use both and do not plan to banish margarine. It functions as a tool to lower calories in a recipe. It gives me flexibility.

Other foods like light mayo are permanent adoptions. I would quit eating mayo rather than switching back to full calorie mayo because it is not worth its weight in calories. I would make homemade mayo, but I eat little mayo. My biggest surprise is that mustard can substitute for it. Now my use of mayo is a choice, not a need.

I bought dehydrated peanut butter one time and have not bought it since. Peanut butter is loaded with fat - the kind that is good for your body. I would rather they add more fat in than remove it. Before I made the purchase, I knew that, but I thought it might be a handy low-calorie flavoring for my shakes. It was lower but still high in calories. Worse, it lent the taste of sand, not peanut butter to my food. I would only recommend it if it is your own personal light margarine. Even then I would be tempted to dilute homemade peanut butter or explore every possible other avenue that does not result in high calorie sand.

Someone discovers a berry growing off a bush has vitamins in it and they dub it a super food. Others ask if eating it will let them re-gain their high school waist line, grow hair, or gain clearer memory. The fact a food our ancestors were eating since antiquity is a magical super food goes to show what a bad state we are in. I take the opposite view. If it does not possess vitamins, anti-oxidation effects, fiber, or something that does not help my body, then it is not food. It is junk marketed to us.

Without the urges to eat for the fun of it and with my sharper tastes, I can enjoy high calorie healthy foods in moderation. I eat peanut butter made with one ingredient - peanuts. Fruits and vegetables are low calorie and dominate my eating. Moreover, they are loaded with useful nutrients. I look back and laugh. Processed foods scared me, and I was not sure how many of them I would have to eat. But, now, I eat more wholesome than ever before. Too much of anything, olive oil or processed cake frosting is bad for you. That is the bigger concern than if it is processed. Once you leave obesity behind, you can join me in avoiding processed foods, but first you must focus on the calories.

8.5. Keep a Lookout

I had a bottle of lemon juice about to go bad and made it into lemonade. It turned out to be a third fewer calories than fruit juice. I replaced juice with lemonade in my strawberry pineapple smoothie. The success made me explore more uses. My toddler and I have been on a homemade popsicle streak. The lemonade smoothie made for ideal popsicles. Each one came in under twenty calories. It takes six of them before I reach a hundred calories, but I get sick of them before half that amount.

Like every home gardener, I grew summer squash. One day a squash is ready and you can find a use for it. But then the next day, more squash is ready, and you have to find another use for more squash. The cycle continues until you are glad the plant is dead. This year I added it into the food I cooked. First, I added it into my taco recipe. It did not seem a traditional fit. I am not even one for adding squash straight by itself, but it tasted like it fit. I went on to add it into other foods. It became my favorite add-in vegetable. Summer squash is fewer calories than onion, clocking in at sixteen calories per hundred grams. It is a great way to lower the calorie density of a dish. For the first time in the history of home gardeners, I was able to use the summer squash I grew, but it came close at the end of the season.

The fifty calorie per serving light margarine I was buying was re-formulated. The regular version is now fifty calories and the light version is thirty-five calories. Fifty calories per tablespoon was fitting into my meals, so I kept to the same calories and purchased the new regular variety. To this day, I have not tried the lighter version. It is great to know I have another option to reduce calories more if I needed to. But right now, I do not need it. It reminded me that the grocery store is a constant place of change. The different flavors and brands change. This one jumped out at me as I was buying it. Now I keep a look out at the items I buy to see if there are any new kinds out there that I might like better.

My tastes changed during this program in unexpected ways. When I was obese, I called tea dirty water. I hated it because I tried it twenty years ago after a high calorie pop. When I started this program, I saw no appeal in tea because it seemed another high calorie sugar drink. Then my mother gave tea to my son, and he cried for it at home. Grandparents are helpful that way. I knew nothing about tea. I bought a plain box labeled tea and used a calorie-free sweetener. Toddler crisis averted. I tried it too. I did not mind drinking a cup of it but felt no desire for more. Yet, I felt promise. The root of the taste was new, different, and calorie free. Next to the plain box teas sat teas flavored with orange, apple, blueberry, and the other fruits I adore. The flavored teas made me want to drink a half gallon. Now I make tea throughout the week and drink it with dinner. It has replaced diet pop for me. Not too bad for dirty water.

I was making a chicken sandwich. The chicken breast marinated overnight in a jerk flavor sauce and cooked on my outdoor hard wood grill. The bun was my homemade sourdough bread. From my garden, I picked tomatoes and jalapeños to add to the sandwich. When I picked up the mayo from the fridge, I paused. It felt like I was about to take a painter's brush to my Picasso and erase the flavors I had worked hard to create. I put the mayo back and got the mustard out. The sandwich screamed with flavor. I never sat out to eat without mayo. Nor did I have too. One tablespoon of light mayo per sandwich fits in my calorie goals. That is how I rode into the healthy weight range. But after that day, eating mayo is now a decision I make, not a requirement. Knowing that feels as good as eating an apple.

At the grocery store, yogurt came in colorful packages plastered with health claims. Many had candy crumbles to mix in. How can I turn down food that comes with candy crumbles? Thus, I tried it. The candy crumbles were everything I expected, but the yogurt part went to the trash. When I started this program, I examined yogurt again. Compared to the ice cream with candy crumbles, the yogurt was still a calorie bargain. I set out to try a different flavor of yogurt each week. No matter the candy flavor, I did not like the yogurt part. I never forced myself to eat it, only to try it. One day, a new kind was on sale. It was the proverbial being in the right place at the right time. I discovered what had tripped me on the other yogurts.

Most yogurt at the grocery store is made from skim milk. This lets them put a low calorie count on it, but is laughable. It comes packaged with full calorie candy crumbles. This new variety that caught my attention was two percent fat yogurt. I could taste the difference. Many people think fat is the enemy, but fat brings a satiety and flavor. Moreover, this kind was not candy crumble flavored, but strawberry flavored. I worked this new yogurt brand into my breakfast. In a few months, it proved my gateway yogurt. I went on to try other yogurt brands. In the end, I learned to make my own homemade yogurt. I mix that with frozen fruit and enjoy as a staple item in my breakfast.

One pound at a time, the journey changed my tastes and outlook on food. What tasted good at first, does not taste good now. Substitution that seemed crazy, like mustard for mayo, are ones I do now but were beyond my comprehension at the start. The flavors and brands change at the grocery store. Different fruits and vegetables are coming in and out of season. I included many examples of foods with the techniques. But, remember to keep a look out for both the food and how you are responding to it. It will not be the same from one month to the next as both you and everything around you is changing.

Chapter 9: Exercise

"Physical fitness is not only one of the most important keys to a healthy body, it is the basis of dynamic and creative intellectual activity." - John F. Kennedy

9.1. New Ways to Hurt Yourself

When I cleared weeds out of my garden on the weekend, I recovered with a trip to the buffet. Mowing the grass merited two fat man-sized cheeseburgers with matching fries and mayo. A ten minute walk earned ten minutes worth of ice cream. As with calories in food, I had no concept of the relative calories burned in exercise. The correct amount is closer to saying an hour walk burns five seconds worth of ice cream. When I flirted with exercise, the calorie estimates are why it never worked for me. It is a danger to start exercising because it is far more work than the extra food you get out of it.

In the first month, I was not ready to exercise, but I felt obliged. Commercials for healthy food show people running, so I assumed that is what healthy people do. I tried to run from the front door to the first tree in the yard. I made it to the first weed. My knees ached, and I was out of breath. It took an hour to recover. The next day I tried again. The second day I made it to the second weed patch. I felt proud I pushed myself, but it took two days to recover. Running was not for me.

Next, I tried work out videos. But, I did not know which workout videos to choose. There were many videos from self proclaimed fitness gurus. I went with them because they looked liked they fit the TV icon image. The gurus claimed thirty minutes of intensity a few times a week would shed the pounds. When I exercised along, I learned an improvement on running. Jumping Jacks allowed me to hurt both my knees and arms at the same time. With pushups, I hurt my elbows, stomach, and back. In the end, I learned new ways to hurt myself and break furniture. The workout videos went to the bottom of my DVD rental queue.

Yet, I was losing one percent of my body weight each week from paying attention to food alone. I pushed the images of five mile hikes out of my head. I came back to the food and focused on it. Everything with food was a different approach than I had taken my whole life. It merited being my top priority.

After three months in, I thought about increasing my physical activity. It was from a feeling of curiosity and not as an obligation. Even then, I did not want to join my local gym and embark on the abs of steel program. Rather, I wanted to move more. Moreover, I did not want to lose weight faster but improve my lifestyle. Those feelings are how I knew I was ready. If you do not have those, then do not be in a rush to add more movement into your life. Also, in that time I had lost over twenty pounds. That would not let me run a marathon, but would let me walk more.

Every morning I waited for the elevator. One day they were doing maintenance to the elevators and just one was operational. There was a big group of others waiting too. I started to check email on my phone. After getting through two dozen emails, there was still no elevator. I wondered if there was someone I could call to complain. The one thing I never wondered was should I take the stairs instead.

When I got home that day, I ordered a pizza, and they said it would be fifty minute wait. I told them no thanks and called another place. The best I found was a forty minute wait, but I spent ten minutes in calling places. With candy in hand, I kicked back on the couch with the TV until the pizza arrived. By the time the pizza got there, I was starved and ate until it was gone. The whole time I felt victimized without a choice. The thought did not cross my mind that I could cook something quicker than the fifty minute wait.

Being fat did not stop me from being able to take the stairs or cook. Those choices were open to me back then. Instead it made me not want to do consider them as options, like a fog of fat clouded my thoughts. I could have done my own anti-workout video on avoiding physical activity. But, I looked through the fog and thought about my day, looking for opportunities to move more. The elevators, pizza, and many others came to mind. Instead I started to look at my life and examine the places where I could move more.

9.2. At Work

I drove to work for forty minutes, sitting the whole time. When I got to work, I used to sit morning to evening except for bathroom breaks. I felt charged in the morning, but by the end of the day felt like a low battery. I assumed that was the nature of a modern job, so I never questioned it. Now, even if I do not have time to go anywhere, I try to stand up from my chair at least once an hour. If I can spare a minute, I walk down the hallway, stairs, or to the other end of the building.

When I was obese, I used the stairs at work during a fire drill because they shut off the elevators. But during the program, I gave the upward direction a try. The first time I went up, I paused every five steps. If someone zipped by while I was resting on the stairs, I pulled out my cell phone and pretended to be checking something. That was not common because most others do not take the stairs. When I made it to the third floor, I looked forward to a day of sitting. I was out of breath but not hurt like in the fitness videos. I walked past the elevator bay trying to project the "I walked up the stairs and you did not attitude." It is one I am still working on. At first, I took the stairs up twice a week and progressed to everyday. Every week I lost more weight, so every week I had to lift less on the stair climb. I was slow at first, but now I can zip up the stairs faster than someone taking the elevator.

Moreover, I make excuses to visit other floors, so I get a chance to use the stairs. Is not the water cooler one floor up better? It is after you had to walk up the stairs to get to it. The best thing that helps me stay focused during a workday is to take a Pac-Man trip through the building. Down the stair well, across the floor, up the other stair well, adding a few zigzags. It is like being in Pac-Man. My prize is a power pill's worth of renewed focus. The days I can do that multiple times are my most productive days at work.

I have to climb to the third floor, but what if you are up higher? There was a local business lunch event I used to go to each month. It was held at a hotel conference room on the tenth floor. This was back when I was in 2x shirts. Still, I broke as soon as I could and made my way to the elevator to ensure I could get out first. One day, I ended up getting involved in a conversation with others after lunch. When I went to leave, there were sixty people in front of me to take an elevator that could hold ten. I had another appointment later that day. A few brave souls declared they were taking the stairs. I joined like a lemming and headed down with them. Any other time, I associate going down stairs with being easy, but it felt like I was trekking through the wild. I took pauses every half floor. At the bottom, I felt like I completed a wilderness hike. But, I had enough energy to walk to my car a block away. If I had been there every day, I would have started by going down the stairs twice a week. Going up that many would require being in shape. But, I would take the first two or three floors by stairs, and then switch over to the elevator for the rest of the way.

9.3. At Home

I sit for forty minutes on the drive home from work. Then I sit at home to watch TV, use the computer, or write this book. I used to record TV shows then fast forward through the commercials. Now I take breaks during the show and spend longer than if it was live. I check my email, drink water, let the dogs out, do a few dishes, or see how many stars are out in the sky. In the obese days, many of my TV breaks were food breaks. I had to combat that problem. First, I kept track of calories so I knew if I could afford to have the potato chips during the commercial. I started to shift into not eating while watching TV, except for popcorn. For instance, I have not eaten pizza and watched TV at the same time in two years. Even when I do have popcorn with TV, I make the popcorn before the show starts and bring it in to eat from the start of the TV show. Then I do not refill the food while watching. With that risk out of the way, my TV breaks are breaks from sitting. And while I do not watch that much TV as compared to playing on the computer, the same applies to that as well.

If I could have found a similar house without a second story, I would be living there now instead. But today as at work, I look for opportunities to use the stairs. I have put a few things on the second floor to give me an excuse to use the stairs more often. Other times I walk up and down them for the fun of it. The staircase is the best exercise equipment I ever purchased.

Moreover, there is a world of more choices for things to do at home than at work. For instance, I do not have a good outdoor walking trail at work, but I do at home. Thus, at home I often walk outside. I do that more than the stairs at home because it adds variety and I like being out in the sun. I may play with the dogs outside or pick up sticks. From mowing the grass to landscaping work, I can find something to do outside. Sometimes I walk to the mailbox instead of checking it when I am coming home from work in my car. This gets me moving and leaves me feeling like I accomplished something.

Moreover, every household chore I have put off offers a movement opportunity. It is amazing how many times I can walk by an unorganized box. After a few times, it blends in to become part of the furniture. Now I go through some of them. I admit to my wife's chagrin that there are still boxes of stuff that was important to me one or two decades ago that still needs to be organized. However, I have gotten many of the others. I even wash dishes if I get desperate for something to do. The act of cooking has become a hobby for me. I get full control over engineering the calories in the food, and I get moving across the kitchen - a true double-win activity. I used to cook when I was obese, but less often and less complicated meals. Now every Sunday is like a mini-Thanksgiving dinner.

9.4. At Hobby

My garden is more square footage than most houses. In the spring time, I prepare the land, put up trellises, and plant. Then onto weeding, more planting, and tending to the plants. I do not have to walk far in the garden to find something that can be done. With the sun shining and temperature pleasant, I spend the entire day working outside. Even after I finish everything that needs to be done, I can find something more to do. On those days, I burn at least a box of ice cream calories, but the extra calories are not the main reason I do it. I do it because I enjoy it. It my hobby and different from my day job, so I get a break from everything else.

Last year my oldest was two years old and ready to "Help Dada" as he puts it. He cried to be a part of what I was doing. It was limited in what he could do, but I worked him in where I can. He helped pull up the onions and put them into buckets. He was my back-up expert at telling which blackberries are ripe. His seven year old cousin visited and did not know which ones were ripe, but he did. This makes it even less like work. Some days running after him adds to my calories burned so I get a box and a half of ice cream calories, but again, it is not the driver.

If I do not work in the garden on the weekend, I like to go somewhere and walk. I have invested in year-long passes to the local zoo and museum. It is the best investment I make. Both are kid friendly and give me opportunities to walk. Once I told someone how often I went to the zoo. They said it seemed boring to go often enough to merit a membership pass. I asked what they did. They muttered something about watching TV and playing video games. I will not find a new life experience on the TV. It is not like they invited a new character type or plot. I know too I will not have a life-altering experience at the zoo next time either. But, I will be the smallest bit healthier for the walk. I will see how the leaves and animals are doing with the sun shining on me. For me, that is the opposite of boring. If you do not have a zoo or museum, then look for a park, walking trial, or large store that offers walking opportunities. Anywhere to give you a chance to walk.

Someone was describing the football playoffs to me. They used terms that did not register with me. Then they mentioned Bengals. I thought they meant the old "Walk Like an Egyptian" music group and asked what concert they were talking about. Turns out there is a football team named that too. I have never been much into sports. But I look forward to playing them with my kids as they get older. It will get me moving in new ways. Anything I can do for recreation that involves moving away from the TV and computer is a win. Even if it means learning new terms.

9.5. Into Exercise

When I started, I thought my end goal would be to get up each morning, run a mile, bench press 300 pounds, have a protein shake, go to work, visit the gym during lunch, come home, and repeat my morning routine. The perfect TV picture of what it means to be in shape. My current goal is to work in exercise that does not feel like exercise and avoid other TV picture views on life. It is the everyday opportunities at work, at home, and within my hobbies that are the best physical activity options. Even if I never lift a weight or run, I still count myself a success at physical activity. Thus, you do not have to feel ready for the next level if you quit living like a sloth. Of course, after a hundred or so pounds gone, you may feel ready for more. I still suggest using more focus as an outgrowth of the prior steps.

Walking can be turned into an exercise routine with a specific goal. Any new cell phone worth its data plan can track your steps. I use mine to track my steps. Many like to throw out a ten thousand per day step goal. I walk up and down three flights of stairs three times per day and do not make that goal. You do not go from a hundred steps per day to ten thousand per day. That is a great way to discourage yourself. I suggest starting smaller, a hundred step goal, a thousand step goal, and more over time. Or, you can do what I do and measure in terms of activity, like using the stairs three times a day or walking half the zoo or the whole zoo. Focusing on walking more is a natural outgrowth.

There is no end to the low-impact exercises you can do. Bicycling and roller blading are not more stressful than walking and give variety and ability to go further distances. A bike trial has pleasant looking scenery. Sports like golf will get you moving, leaving you feeling like you did a hobby, and gentle enough on your body that old guys play the sport professionally. Then you can get into other activities from hobby-based, like dancing, through to actual exercise like water aerobics. The whole world is open to you. Start with the ones which are low-impact and natural outgrowths of things you enjoy to do.

Yoga is the one exercise that is not a hobby I do. Even then it is sort of a hobby. I have done it off and on since I was a teenager, but more off than on in the last decades. Yoga offers a range from low-impact I could do even when I was extremely morbidly obese to power yoga routines that leave me feeling like I ran a marathon.

The best benefit is not physical at all. I had a new high stress project at work. Every time I sat or laid down, I thought over what could go wrong at work, what I needed to do, or what I was overlooking. The challenge at work felt right. I was doing well and wanted to succeed at it. But I knew if I could not relax when not at work or at least sleeping that I would not be successful for longer. I remembered yoga from years back and started doing it again. The first night, my mind felt silent for the first time in months and I could sleep. That project was a major success and one I look back on with pride. I have since gone onto even more challenging ones.

Beyond stress relief, the light forms of yoga do not burn many calories. They get you moving, build muscle tone, and flexibility. If you want your body to look better, muscle tone will do it. Even if you are overweight, yoga tones what muscle you have. The added flexibility will prepare you for other exercises. As I mentioned, the biggest problem with exercising when you are obese is hurting yourself. As you progress, you can try out power yoga for other benefits, but do not rush it. There are other exercises like yoga you can find with similar characteristics. I suggest you find what you like.

As I lost weight, more thoughts came to me. I have lived in the same town for years, but I never noticed all the 5k marathons until last summer. Every little attraction has its own sort of marathon. My town does, the neighboring town does and the local apple orchard sponsors one. I am sure they had signs up for these events the years before, but the fog of fat let me overlook them. It was not until the end of the season I noticed them all. I could not do one this last year, but I am planning on trying one in the future.

High-cardiovascular exercise, like aerobics, gardening, and bicycling get your heart rate up and can burn enough calories for an extra dinner or two. Most summer weekends, I burn over a thousand net calories working in my garden. If you are looking for a way to eat tons more calories in a day, then that is the way. However, this news has a downside. When your single goal is to earn more food calories, it feels like work and is not enjoyable. I have taken laps around the yard to balance the calories for indulgent food I wanted to have. Not one of those times after I ate did I think it had been worth it. Now if I burn those calories because I was doing things I enjoy, then I do feel good about eating later. Moreover, sometimes I get sick of having to eat to recover the calories. When I am doing physical activity for long periods, I run down my batteries. The feeling is like being tired. Then I eat and recharge and I am ready to go more. It feels like your body is a machine that runs on fuel, which it is. But it felt strange at first since I used to look at food for fun and not a fuel.

At the other end, strength training does not burn enough calories for an extra dinner. You might get an extra snack. But, it will give you something exotic - a higher base burn rate. The more muscle your body has, the more calories it burns doing nothing. Thus, as you strength train, you build muscle and your base calories go up. However, it is a slow process. The extra calories will not be there until long after you want them. By that time, you will be used to fewer calories. If I was looking to eat more, I would focus more on strength training to increase my base because I feel like I have reached a good point with food intake. Beyond the calories gained, you get better body definition and strength. Do it enough and you can become one of the body builders that pay attention to the BMI scale. Of course, only do strength training if you enjoy it.

9.6. Tracking Calories

Remember the calorie deficit between what your body burns doing nothing and how much you eat? If you are physically active, then your body burns more base calories. It is equivalent to eating less and creating a larger-than-intended calorie deficit. The same risk of going too low on calories is there. Simple light moving around is not a concern, but heavier physical activities become important to track.

At first, I was not trying to do extra physical activity. Then we had a snow storm. I spent over a half-hour shoveling snow. I ate a normal dinner, but felt like I had not eaten. Using an online calculator, I discovered that shoveling snow burns meal level calories. At the other end, when I first started tracking steps, I thought I would discover another meal's worth of calories. It turned out to be rounding error level when I started. Any physical activity that takes more than five minutes and leaves you feeling out of breath is the sort of thing to start considering for calories burned. Most activities are low, so there is not much of risk of accidentally forgetting about it. Strenuous things like shoveling snow, you know you did. If you do something unexpected like shovel snow, and feel empty after eating your normal amount, then look it up.

When counting calories from exercise, be aware of net burned calories. The treadmill will say you burned sixty calories from a twenty-five minute work out, but you would have burned fifty calories if you had sat on the couch instead. Your body burns calories doing nothing. Most exercise calorie charts and digital equipment will include the base because a higher number leaves you feeling like you accomplished more. Most step trackers will do so likewise. A few by default will give you net calories. Be sure to check because it makes a big difference.

Of course, not everything has a treadmill calorie display. For normal activities there are reference charts and online calculators that can use your basic information, time spent, and type of activity to give a ballpark estimate. A good mobile app for tracking calories should have this integrated. You need to make sure you are honest on the time spent and ensure you are counting net, not gross, calories. These online reference charts can have errors, but they are a good ballpark.

For normal daily activity, like walking, there are activity and step trackers. Newer cell phones can track your steps, and today many of us are glued to our cell phones. I use mine to track my steps.

Whenever I do heavy cardio activity, other than walking, like gardening or lots of cooking, I use a heart rate monitor (HRM). It tells me the calories burned based on my heart rate. Mine even has a happy birthday message each year on my birthday. It is second to my cell phone for most useful personal electronic device.

If you look for a HRM, I recommend the two part kind. These have a strap that goes around your chest. That device broadcasts your heart rate to a receiver, like a watch or a cell phone. There are HRMs that work off your wrist alone, but they are not as accurate. As technology improves, they may get there. Of course, if you do not do much heavy cardio and mainly walk, such a device may be better for you.

I do not bother to use my HRM if I am doing something minor that will not burn that many calories. When I started, I did not know what those activities were, but I had a chance to use the HRM doing everything and learned which things are. Do not forget many chores burn calories. Cooking a large meal in the kitchen burns calories. Every Saturday morning I burn at least fifty calories doing various food preparation activities for breakfast and the rest of the day. If you are not sure, these things double on the list of chores you have been avoiding or the ones most on your spouse's honey-do list. For walking, even at the zoo, I use the step tracker built into my cell phone because it is easy.

9.7. Spending It

After the first few months, moving was part of my lifestyle. Beyond that, can exercise calories be part of a regular planned calorie deficit? When I had over a hundred pounds to lose, the answer was no. At that weight, I was cut off from most exercise options. Even though I had my gardening I could only do heavy activities once or twice a week. I was not in shape to do it regularly through the week. I was best off trying to add movement in my day. When I earned extra calories, I viewed them as random presents to eat more that day. I believe in focusing on the food first. Before this program, when I did physical activity, I ate back twice the calories. Now I eat back one to one.

Once you are not obese, then regular exercise can be part of your calorie deficit plan to ride into your target weight. Do not feel like it has to be, but you have the choice. To get to that weight, you had to master food. Being that much lighter opens exercise options to you and removes the fog of fat in considering physical activity. I am content with my current calories and weight, but if I wanted to drop a few more pounds, I would focus on exercising down.

Today I was finishing up installing a laminate floor in one of my rooms. The HRM showed over a thousand calories net burned. I added an extra item into each meal that day. Between the meals I added fruit and a bowl of mixed veggies with cream butter. After dinner I had three sourdough cinnamon rolls with cream cheese glaze. I am still under and need to eat more. Fear the Walking Dead comes on tonight. I may watch it with buttered popcorn. The calories you gain from exercising are yours to do with as you wish. Two years ago, I would have plowed today's calories into a carton of ice cream. Part of what you prefer to do with those extra calories changes over time. When I am working in the garden in spring, I may add a second lunch or dinner. Other times I play it strategic and plan for an indulgent choice. I try to line up planned heavy burn days with the pizza from the local pizzeria.

There have been other days when I have been active the entire day in a big outdoor project. I eat throughout the day. At the end of the day, I am still under and have to seek out more to eat. I get sick of having to eat more. Looking for more calories to eat was never something I needed to do when I was obese, but now I have to think about it. It is hard to eat an avalanche of calories when your go to snacks are fruit, mixed veggies, and popcorn. But, every other day of the year, when I am trying to avoid eating too much instead of not enough, those low calorie snacks help.

Gaining extra calories from exercise sounds like ice cream with sprinkles. It may tempt you to jump into exercise sooner or over do it. But, there will never be enough calories for everything you can dream up. That is why I was obese to start with. I kept wanting more. Exercise will give you more calories, but remember it is about living within your means.

Chapter 10: Parting Plans

"The future belongs to those who believe in the beauty of their dreams."
- Eleanor Roosevelt

10.1. Adjusting Calories

I calculated a calorie goal target and plunged in. The start was a new way of approaching life. I did not concern myself by how far my calorie goal would have to drop to reach the target weight I wanted to be at in five years. I concerned myself with starting to lose a few pounds. After three months and over twenty pounds gone, I felt comfortable in my new approach. At that point, I looked at how my calorie goal would have to progress. The same five hundred calorie deficit at three hundred pounds would maintain my weight at two hundred fifty pounds. As I lost weight, my body needed to burn fewer calories doing nothing, since there was less fat to maintain. To continue my weight loss, I lowered my calorie goal as I went. The most important thing was to start the journey, not to worry about a calorie goal months out.

I calculated the base calories I burned at my current weight and at my ideal five year target weight. I revisited those numbers every month, but I did not change them each month. When I was comfortable, I did minor adjustments to keep my weight loss goal on track. Then not too long in, I reached the point where a thousand calories per day separated the maintenance level for my current weight and target weight. That is the same as a two pound per week rate. I took that as my goal and rode it to where I am today. During that ride, I let go of aiming for an amount per week. It was two pounds per week at first. After a few months, it was a pound and three quarters each week and continued to slow from there.

In particular, I did not aim for a calorie goal less than my ideal weight. I could have reached target weight a few months earlier if I had, and maybe you would be reading this book a few months earlier too. But I would have increased my risk of falling off the wagon and getting stuck above my target weight.

How do you cope with eating fewer calories? If you ask that question and visualize food disappearing from your plate, then it is not time to ask that question. In the end, no one will care if you lost a pound per week instead a pound and a half per week. Reduce once you feel comfortable with your current goal, not before.

There is nothing that says you have to keep reducing calories. You will have to stop when you reach target weight. You could take your initial calorie goal and ride it until weight loss stops. After a few months of no weight loss, you can decide what you want to do. You will be making decisions with less fog of fat and a history of success behind you.

In contrast, if you feel good about your new lifestyle and are ready to continue weight loss, then read on. It is a game of knowledge that you gain experience with as you play. Upfront, I did not know the calorie engineering techniques I outlined. Thus, the discovery and application of new methods let me lower my calorie goal without an impact on what I was eating. For instance, discovering how to make a calorie sensible hamburger was a moon step forward. Even when I knew a technique, I did not realize how I could apply it. At first, it was crazy talk to replace an over-sized bun with two slices of light bread. Then one day I was doing it. I outlined many techniques with examples. Do not apply all of them at once. Use only what you need to get the starting calorie goal. Then once you lose twenty pounds, apply more of techniques to continue. And, sometimes it is a matter of looking at the technique in a new light and realizing that it applies more broadly than you realize. My words will not change the second time you look over the techniques, but you will have changed. I highlighted the food I ate as examples. What you eat may be different or change in your own journey. But, the same techniques apply to all foods.

Thinking of calories as a range between target weight loss per week and maintaining my weight helped. When I went to shift down calories, I would phase it over a month by starting to aim for the lower end of the range each day. After a few weeks, I had narrowed my calorie range and did not miss it. I debated about offering more tips on coping with stepping down, but once I hit the last thousand calorie difference I quit reducing. The first problem is to start. The second is a small period where you do reduce calories. Then the rest of learning to live with an amount that will take you to target weight and keep you there. Enjoy the journey and get started.

10.2. When to Stop

When I started my journey, my dream weight was one hundred eighty pounds. I put that in as my goal in my calorie tracker mobile app. One day I updated my weight, and my daily calorie goal increased. It was telling me to eat more to gain back weight back up to one hundred eighty pounds. I laughed. From the BMI categories, my healthy weight range is one hundred forty to one eighty eight pounds. If I wanted, I could hit the lower end of that range or even go under it. But where would it end?

A lifetime of feeling fat does not go away when the fat goes away. I thought it would, but it does not. No matter what the scale said, what size my clothes were, or what my wife said, I felt fat every pound of the way. When I crossed into the healthy weight range, I kept reminding myself that I was in the target range. It took six months of being in that range for the fat feeling to start to fade. Then more months after that for my subconscious to quit self identifying as fat.

I quit reducing my daily calorie goal long before I hit the top of healthy weight range. Thus, I was not losing much each week by that point. It gave my mind time to catch up to my body. If I plowed into the range at two pounds per week, I might be writing from a hospital bed. The feeling of being fat goes away, but it takes more time than the pounds do.

I read about a woman who was trying to recover from anorexia. She did not have the energy to walk. The doctors were concerned that if they raised her calories anymore than twenty five per day that it might kill her. Twenty five calories is less than half a cookie. If I cannot walk due to my weight, I would rather be at the opposite end of the spectrum. Neither is healthy and both will kill you. But if I am stuck in bed due to my weight, I would rather be stuck in bed with a happy meal than a feeding tube.

Once I hit the BMI overweight category, I received suggestions from others. They warned me about not having muscle, being too thin, or offered candy. I appreciated the concern, but it felt odd to begin to get it before I was in the healthy weight range. Overweight is the normal for our age, and that what others were judging me against. Being overweight is now considered normal by most. I never fit in with the crowd when I was extremely morbidly obese. With the general population heading to where I was, it was good I moved out of danger of being like everyone else.

Over a year ago, I set my daily calorie goal to the maintenance weight for 180 pounds. During the time I narrowed in, I knew the weight I was headed towards. In fact, I landed a few pounds under my target weight. And with daily fluctuations, I am in the range.

To start this journey, I listed reasons to change my lifestyle. I compared my weight to those reasons. The reasons were for me to start, but the same reasons let me know when to end. If I was twenty pounds heavier or lighter, would I be able to run with my children? The answer would be no, so I know I am in the right range.

10.3. Tracking Progress

My wife keeps a clock in the bathroom. She says it has sentimental value from before we met. It tells me the phase of the day more than the time of the day. The second hand skips a few seconds, falls behind a few seconds, and makes wild jumps. Sometimes it even has the right time of another time zone. It belongs in the bathroom because I cannot think of a better companion for the bathroom scale.

If I weighed myself before going to bed, then the next morning, the number was a surprise. In my sleep, I may have gained or lost five pounds. If I waited ten minutes and re-weighed myself, it shifted again. I tried exhaling before I weigh myself, leaning different directions, and trying to will the number from my mind to the scale. None of that works. In the short term, the scale is in a mood and destined to display what it wants. It does not help that a weight loss goal is two pounds or less per week, and that is within the error swing.

To combat the moodiness of the scale, I planned to weigh myself once a week. I ended up weighing myself every other day. I dreamed of seeing a steady procession of tenths of a pound every day. Instead, every random number of days, I would be about two pounds lighter. When the number surprised me, I would not record it. Instead, I weighed myself the next few days in a row until I got the answer I thought was right. After that, I would try to go another week until another weigh in. After a few weeks of progress, I was comfortable with longer pauses between weigh-ins and did not need to keep weighing each day to shop for a number.

But with the numbers all over the place, how did I know what was right and what to ignore? I looked over the last four weeks and averaged it across the weeks. When I looked this way, it was a downhill curve without peaks. As I got into my current weight, I could see my weight loss decreasing to fractions of a pound. Then my weight stabilized about the same number range month to month. That is how I know I was done with losing weight.

I would go a few months and then out of nowhere my pants were in danger of falling down. I checked my belt and reined in one more notch. The shoulders in my shirt looked big in the mirror. My wife would confront me and tell me my clothes were too big. I avoided clothes shopping because I needed to go every month to keep up. The first thing I had to do was try on clothes to learn my new size. That was much like the obese days, but I used to discover how high the pant sizes went. Now I discovered how low they went. No curve on the weight graph ever gave me as much enjoyment as when I passed from the big size section to the regular size section for pants. For as much as I avoided clothes shopping, once I went, it felt like being at a calorie free pizza buffet.

Looking myself in the mirror each day did not provide any signs of progress. But when I compared pictures of myself from month to month, I would stare and ask my wife "Why did not you tell me I was that fat?" I started posing for a picture at least once a month. When we went to the local zoo, I would pose on the bridge in front of the bear and have my wife take a picture. I compared the picture to the prior months and marveled at how thin I looked. Then a few months later, I thought I looked big in the prior picture. If I had it to do over again, I would have taken a selfie each week I weighed myself. A history of scale numbers makes a graph, but a history of pictures tells a story.

My food journal was a log of everything I was eating and drinking with calories. I rechecked the base calories my body burns doing nothing and compared to my food journal average. It was the elegance of engineering. The math was solid; the journal was accurate; I did not need to worry. Every few weeks I looked over receipts from the grocery store and dining out and ask if those kinds of foods were logged. It was not a perfect audit, but it provided an external check. Once I was doing my journal for a few weeks, I knew if I was keeping it up-to-date or not.

In the obese days, I was losing two or more pounds per week and felt better every month. I quit feeling like I needed an aspirin every day. Sleeping through the night became regular. The changes were too small to notice each day except as I remember back to how I felt. But the energy I gained was noticeable in other ways. When I did a task I had not done in awhile, like pickup tree branches, it went faster than I remembered from before. Moreover, I had energy to go on and do more things. I used to go to the buffet after gathering tree branches because I was so exhausted, but now I had the energy to cook dinner after.

10.4. The Hunger

Keeping an eating schedule makes eating a habit. After you spend weeks and months in a set eating routine, it is the rare day when you feel hungry outside that routine. On the other hand, if you slip in random mini-meals or skip meals, then you will put my book aside. If I have a meeting, family trip, or something else that knocks aside my schedule, I adjust. But I do my best to stick to it. If you find yourself getting hungry between meals, then the schedule is too long, the calorie goal is too aggressive, the food has too much sugar, or all of these things. Check and fix each aspect in turn, starting with the calorie goal.

Before I started, I was eating two third-pound cheeseburgers loaded with enough mayo to count as another burger. When I started this program, I ate a single quarter-pound cheeseburger for dinner. I was hungry afterward and went on to eat ice cream to help fill the void. It was too big of a step at first. Even today at target weight, I eat two cheeseburgers for dinner, plus a snack after dinner. Thus, I focused on getting the mayo down below the level of another hamburger. That was a good enough step to start with. Hungry often means you are taking too big of a step at once.

Roast chicken with mashed potatoes, gravy, and corn is one of my favorite meals. It has enough variety and amount to satisfy a recovering obese person. However, when I first started, I set a reasonable calorie goal for dinner and ate. After a single plateful, I felt hungry. I ate up until the calories need to maintain my current weight and craved more. I had no judgment of what hunger meant. When I was obese, a satisfying meal meant my stomach was stuffed and could not hold more. That was my eating guide. Now that I have lost the weight, my hunger feeling is like a car feels on empty. Sometimes I confuse whether I am tired or I need to eat more because the feelings are close. I started to trust my food journal and use the calories to maintain my weight as a ceiling. Except if there was a day when I did physical exercise, like shoveling the snow. Otherwise, part of this program was learning what hunger feels like.

At the start, my body was like a car with a dysfunctional fuel gauge. I could not trust it when it came to food. As I lost weight and became closer to ideal weight, those systems started working. I am not saying not to listen to your body, but you need to take it with a "grain of fat". Are you pushing too aggressive of a calorie deficit, or are you not used to eating the calories to maintain your weight?

A single pizza can pack enough calories for a whole day's allowance. Yet it is one of my favorite foods. When I eat one slice, I feel ready for another slice, until there are not anymore slices to tempt me. If while eating I talk to my family, get up from my chair and take a short walk, or do anything to slow myself down, then I am satisfied with less than half of the pizza. Pausing and eating slower helps with the hunger.

I want to add a disclaimer to this particular tip. A hundred pounds ago, it felt like there was no amount of time of waiting and feeling full. However, as I came down from very severely obese to just obese, I began to notice this effect. At a healthy weight, I get the pizza full feeling during the meal. The more you weigh, the longer the time it takes to register. That and part of it is learning to tell hunger apart from the feeling of your stomach being stuffed.

My homemade chicken soup is seventy calories per hundred grams. Three giant bowls compromise my dinner. I feel stuffed like the old days and have calories left over. In contrast, take deep fried popcorn chicken. I ate it like it was movie popcorn and never felt stuffed. But, I spent two days worth of calories on it. Thus, if I do not feel content after eating, I ask myself is it me or is it the food? I try to avoid non-satisfying foods or at least eat them less often.

Sometimes hunger hits more as a deserve-a-food feeling. There were days when I felt like I deserved the death by chocolate torte dusted with powdered sugar. But, I felt like I deserved not get heart disease and have everything I listed as a reason for why I am doing this program. I was right on both. When those two feelings come together I know which one is more important. But I know I cannot live a life of having to choose between two right things every day. Thus, I cut the sugar in the torte, made smaller serving sizes, or replaced it outright with another dessert. Taking a food and engineering the calories to fit through the techniques I have given is a foundation of calorie engineering. I can make and have my torte without the heart disease risk.

Other times hunger is a feeling to eat enough to run a buffet kitchen out-of-stock. The urge goes away with time. The closest I get today is an urge to eat a higher calorie food, like pizza. But, that advice is not much help in the beginning. Fortunately, I remember my old friend of gluttony. What I did was focus on lower calorie density foods. Stews, chili, and anything else that came in under a hundred calories per hundred grams. I can be a glutton on those and still have calories left over. Other times I would plan to do one of my hobby activities, like gardening, that burned gluttony level calories. For instance, I knew from experience that tilling a garden plot and other activities gave me enough calories to have anything I wanted. Thus, I do those activities when I want the deep dish pizza with popcorn chicken. Part of why that works is that I am already going to be doing those activities at some point and know how many calories they will be. If you just say general exercise, then there is nothing that will make you do it. And as I mentioned, most exercises do not burn enough calories to cover gluttony level urges.

10.5. When You Slip

The first key is not to plan to slip. I do not wake up to a day expecting it to be a free day. A binge eating habit is as healthy as a binge drinking habit. On the holidays, I stay on guard, plan, and do extra exercise. I try to be the one preparing the food because I can burn a meal worth of calories over a day of holiday food preparation. Traveling out of town is harder than the holidays for me. It is more work to watch calories dining out. Doing that for every meal in a town where many of the restaurants are foreign to me takes skill. But, even that I am better at navigating today with practice.

When I slipped the first day, I was tempted to make it up tomorrow. But waking up to a day with negative calories would be like waking up to news that the Walking Dead was canceled. Even if I did borrow forward, when tomorrow arrived, I would have to borrow from the next tomorrow. Every day I would feel like I was being punished. Until I had borrowed a month's worth of calories, then I would have given up. Thus, I do not do borrow calories between days. Despite my advice, if you still want to do it, then I suggest you lend forward instead of borrowing from tomorrow. Under eat today because tomorrow is Thanksgiving. You will know how many calories you can go over. It is the difference between using money from savings versus putting it on a credit card.

What do I do if I slip one day? I forget about it. In my mind, I have a perfect score at this game. Each day is an island. When tomorrow comes, it is a new day - one where my favorite TV series has not been canceled. A minor blimp a few times per year is not an issue. The impact is, over the course of two years, it took me a few days longer to get to target weight. I accept that.

On my birthday, I go in prepared to eat up to the calories needed to maintain my current weight. Thus, I planned to let go of the normal calorie deficit for the day. Does that mean I planned to slip? What does it mean to slip? No slip I have ever had in this program equals the height of my former buffet trips. I can eat up to the calories that maintain my current weight with the effect being a pause in weight loss and nothing more. It is not until I go past that level of calories that I start to undo progress. Even then it takes the same calorie surplus to gain it back. Thus, thirty-five hundred calories over the calories to maintain your weight for a week to gain a pound back. Eating that much food in a day is hard. I did it back when I was obese at the buffet trying to get my money's worth. It was hard then too. If your normal days are on track, then it takes determination and focused effort to over eat a huge amount in a week or month.

There is a problem if you are into the program and slipping every week. The start requires dialing in a calorie goal, so slipping will happen. But once you are on your way, you should not slip every week. If this is happening, then it is important to ask why it is happening? My main suspicion is too aggressive of a calorie goal, which will derail the program. If you slip one day in every week, then your average calories for the week are higher than your goal. Raise your daily calorie goal so that you can enjoy every day of the week. You will lose weight on a less aggressive calorie deficit. It will mean going slower, but that is not a bad thing. It took me two years to reach my current weight. What if it had took me four years? I would still have a book to write.

More often I slip within a day for a meal. If it is about a hundred calories, I balance within the day, adjusting the other meals. However, when I have pizza for lunch that guarantees blowing two meals worth of calories. I know from a lifetime of over-eating that I will be hungry later despite one giant meal. There is no making-up a whole extra meal in the day. The temptation becomes to blow the rest of the day since it is already shot. When those meals happen, I treat them as their own mini-islands. I treat it like I ate the regular amount of lunch and move on.

If you fall off the wagon and are picking this book up from under the candy wrappers, then start over. The beauty of this program is that it is repeatable. I do not worry about my weight anymore. If one day I woke up back north of three hundred pounds, I know I did this once and can do it again. Of course, having gone through it and learning everything I learned provides a great deal of insurance of that ever happening.

10.6. Weight of Forever

I was filling-up on gas and noticed the sign for a rewards credit card. It said earn rewards on gas and use in the store to buy a large drink. A stick figure with drink in hand was below the words. Then it said earn even more rewards from that second purchase and suggested you buy candy. The stick figure had a candy bar added. By the end of the sign, the stick figure had a hot dog and pizza. If the stick figure had been a circle figure, that would have been me.

As big as I was, I was not the whole problem. Neither are you. Yet, accepting that part of the problem lay with my choices gave me power. That one small piece, even if one percent, was mine to control. It would have been impossible to start with changing our culture at large, but starting with my own personal choices was possible.

When I started, I feared the life I would have to lead every day, week, month, year, and decade. It was an endless panel of a stick figure passing by candy, hot dogs, and everything else I had lived on. The weight of forever was heavier than I was. I took a deep breath. Then I told myself I can do this today, and I can do this tomorrow. Each day I repeated that message to myself. I focused on today where the battle is at.

It was a new skill to engineer calories. But as I went along, I know the calories in food without thought. When I used to see a donut, I thought "I hope it has sprinkles on it." Now when I see a donut I think three hundred calories. Then I consider if I want to spend that much on a single donut versus something else, like homemade cheesecake.

It is not about building will power. It takes as much will power as when I was obese to turn down homemade pecan pie on Thanksgiving. Did I mention I ate pecan pie last Thanksgiving? It is about shifting into a better lifestyle where everything you do happens without thinking. My old habit would have been eating pecan pie if offered it at breakfast. My new habit would be to decline it as a breakfast option. No thought involved. Moreover, my tastes are sharper. I like a pecan pie based on a custard. I hate the taste of the more common variety that is based on corn syrup. There is no taste temptation for that one. This is a natural reaction not something I have to think about. Last, the urge to eat the whole pie has left with the pounds. My body feedback system for if I have eaten enough started working a few pounds north of healthy weight. I do not have to keep track as closely anymore.

I do now because it helped get me to here and to make sure I do not drift.

The lifestyle change happened one calorie at a time. I could not have woken up one day and approached food like I do today. The time spent losing weight was spent becoming comfortable with a new lifestyle. I never wish that I could eat like I used to. I have eaten enough ice cream in my life to reach Zen five times over, so I know I am not missing anything.

As I came within a few pounds of being healthy weight, I still felt fat. Even after I crossed the threshold, my self image did not change. I had to look down standing up and see how vertical I was. Even then I would have to look down two, three, or ten more times because I could not believe it was me. Even if I had woke up skinny overnight one day, it would have taken two years to accept I was not fat.

If ever I had a doubt about what I was doing, I asked the one person who can never lie to me about anything. The one person whose gaze I can never meet straight on if there is any deceit between us. I see that person in the mirror each day; I am sure you do as well.

The journey does not have to be approached as a harrowing odyssey. It can be fun too. Engineering the calories in the foods I wanted to eat was a rewarding challenge. The same way you feel after solving a tough problem at work. On the lighter side, I found my fighting song for encouragement - "You're the best" from the 1984 Karate Kid movie. If it helps Daniel take on Cobra Kai, then it can help me take on a large sausage pizza.

On the Internet, I see postings from people who want to lose weight but do not want to change the food they eat or anything else. They are looking for a gimmick. The hardest part is the commitment to start. Why change your lifestyle? The math in this program works for the calorie calculations and will let you make fancy graphs showing your progress. None of the math answers the real question of, "Why are you doing this?" During the journey, I came back to my answers.

10.7. The Ritz

"Can you believe it? Your shirt is falling apart after only ten years." - Gina Young

In the winter before I started this program, I bought a black wool coat. Even on sale, it was the most I had ever spent on a coat. By the next winter, it no longer fit. I went back to the place that sold it to me. They said they could not alter it and suggested I buy a new one from them. Instead, I looked up local alterations shops. I took the coat there. They said they would take in the shoulders, bring in the back, and move over the buttons. It sounded like a plan. When I went to pick it up, they asked me for weight loss tips. They wondered if some of their relatives could pull off what I had done. As for the coat, they told me they had to take out enough fabric to make another coat. But in the end, it came out looking like I had bought it in my new size. I wore that coat throughout the winter. The second winter I went back and had a smaller touch-up done. While I was there, I asked about an old leather coat I had. They said leather alteration would cost as much as a new coat to alter and suggested I sell it online and apply it towards a new one. Good news though, I got a great after Christmas deal on a new leather coat.

A jacket is expensive and feels personal. Other items were easier to let go. When I do, I donate them. As I started, I rolled through clothes, so most were far better shape than my own body. I hope the next owner likes them as much as I did. Through some random act of coincidence, I hope they find my book.

My approach to getting rid of clothes was to keep one set from the prior phase. I packed the old clothes away, or rather piled boxes up in my bedroom. I did not know how long my journey would last. In the short-term, I could have slipped back into a prior pant size. After I was in this for a few months, I knew I would not be going back to the start. The danger was the short-term.

I had a large collection of clothes from my journey up in weight. Once I started the other direction, I found my favorite old T-shirt. It was blue, with number 79 written on it, filled in with the American flag.

I think I tried it on every three weeks. My wife says multiple times a week, but I do not think I was that bad most weeks. Then a day came when the t-shirt fit again. I wore it working outside, dirtied it well, painted in it, and put a few more holes in it. It was like being reunited with an old childhood friend. Then the day came when it was too big. By that point, it had had taken more wear and tear than a shirt was ever meant to. With a toast of calorie-free tea, I said goodbye. I thought I threw it away, but the other day I found it in a stack of things. Wearing it is behind me, but maybe I can hang it up in memory. My wife will love that. I almost regret not keeping more old clothes around when I was gaining weight. But truth be told, those clothes are old, and clothes do not age well. It is fun to wear again what you saved. But, it is short trip down memory lane towards your new home on "Healthy Weight Lane".

My mom was cleaning out her house. She found my old high school letterman jacket. It was, for two decades, sitting in a plastic tote waiting for me. I remembered wearing that coat on many nights of activities I hope my kids never do. My old school id, gloves, and enough arcade tokens for a game of Pac-Man were in the pockets. I tried it on. It fit but was a bit big. How many of my old classmates could say the same? I plan on wearing it around one day to see if anyone notices. I might even go to a high school reunion. You cannot go back, but you can take the pounds off.

Appendix

"As far as the laws of mathematics refer to reality, they are not certain, and as far as they are certain, they do not refer to reality." - Albert Einstein

A.1. BMI Scale

See http://WilliamRayYoung.com for online calculators.

Category	BMI Range
Very Severely Underweight	Less than 15
Severely Underweight	From 15 to 16
Underweight	Less than 18.5
Normal Weight	From 18.5 to 25
Overweight	From 25 to 30
Obese Class 1 (Moderately Obese)	From 30 to 35
Obese Class 2 (Severely Obese)	From 35 to 40
Obese Class 3 (Very Severely Obese)	Over 40

To calculate your BMI:
BMI = weight in kilograms / height in meters squared

To find a weight for a target BMI:
Weight in kilograms = BMI * height in meters squared

It felt like being kicked to look at chart that reduced me to a number with an insulting label. My BMI was "over 40" when I started. I invented new category names to amuse myself. Where is "Pleasantly Plump"? How much do I have to lose before I am "Just Fat." When I am starting out at Class 3 Very Severely Obese, "Just Fat" looks like a compliment.

Why then did I bother putting it in the book? As I lost weight, I focused on the next power of ten, going from two-ninety to two-eighty. However, losing ten pounds at two-ninety is not the same as losing ten pounds at two-twenty. The above chart gives you another way to consider your weight. I calculated my weight for each range and those where my longer-term goals during the journey. Moreover, I noticed I felt different at each category. For instance, the urge to eat is different at "Pleasantly Plump" than "Just Fat".

Also, BMI can give you a target weight range. Take the index number for a category, like "Normal Weight", and you can work out what you need to weigh to be in that BMI category. Take the starting and ending index numbers to establish a range. The range for "Normal Weight" was my five year goal when I started.

Every disclaimer of BMI comes with the word average. It does not make any difference if your weight is from muscle or fat. Thus, a body builder is obese by this scale. However, if you are reading this book, then you are not a body builder and do not need to worry.

A.2. Calculate Calories

See http://WilliamRayYoung.com for online calculators.

To lose one pound in a week, you need to eat 3,500 calories less than what your body burns keeping the lights on. This would divide across the seven days in a week to a 500 calorie deficit per day. Listed below is how the weekly deficit works out to a daily deficit.

Pounds Per Week	Weekly Calorie Deficit	Daily Calorie Deficit
½ pound	1,750	250
1 pound	3,500	500
1 ½ pounds	5,250	750
2 pounds	7,000	1,000
2 ½ pounds	8,750	1,250
3 pounds	10,500	1,500

This table is missing one important column - your daily calorie goal. Calculate how many calories your body burns doing nothing and then subtract the amount from the table to find what your daily calorie goal needs to be. Remember not to exceed one percent of your body weight per week. For most people, this means one to two pounds at most per week. But, I started north of three hundred and included three pounds for reference. Also, as you lose weight, the one percent becomes less pounds and calories. It was safe for me to lose three pounds per week in the first few months. After that, I lost less each week as I went, which is the ideal way to do it.

I did not understand why different websites gave me different calories estimates. They could be different by hundreds of calories. The reason is there are multiple formulas to estimate your calories burned. The original is the Harris Benedict equation, and there was a 1984 revised version of it. In 1990, the Mifflin-St. Jeor Equation came out which is what I recommend. Be sure to check what is being used on a website calculator.

To calculate calories burned require two steps. First, you calculate your basal metabolic rate (BMR). This is the number of calories you burn if you laid in bed for a full day. Second, you take that number and apply a multiplier to estimate how often you are out of bed moving around. This is where you can go wrong. Even if you think you are the most active obese person out there, answer sedentary, which will apply a 1.2 multiplier. Add in your exercises ala carte instead of making broad assumptions.

Mifflin-St. Jeor Equation for BMR
For Men
$BMR = 10 * weight + 6.25 * height - 5 * age + 5$
For Women
$BMR = 10 * weight + 6.25 * height - 5 * age - 161$
With weight in kilograms, height in centimeters, and age in years

Calories to maintain your weight $= 1.2 * BMR$
The 1.2 represents sedentary lifestyle. Add calories burnt from exercising to this number.

Once you have a few weeks of weigh-ins, you can figure your actual calories burned based on actual results. That too is an estimate because you weigh less now and may be more or less physically active than the prior weeks. But, it is personalized to you based on your own results.

Calories burned = (weight from four weeks ago - weight today) / 4 weeks / 3500 calories

I like knowing the calories I burn per minute. To calculate take the calories you burn and divide by 1,440, which is the number of minutes in a day. For a long time, my burn rate was about 2 calories per minute. That means in an hour of doing nothing I burn 120 calories. This is handy to subtract from any exercise equipment, like treadmills, that report out gross calories burned.

www.ingramcontent.com/pod-product-compliance
Lightning Source LLC
Chambersburg PA
CBHW050454290526
45786CB00006B/2284